THE
HEALING
POWER
OF
WITCHCRAFT

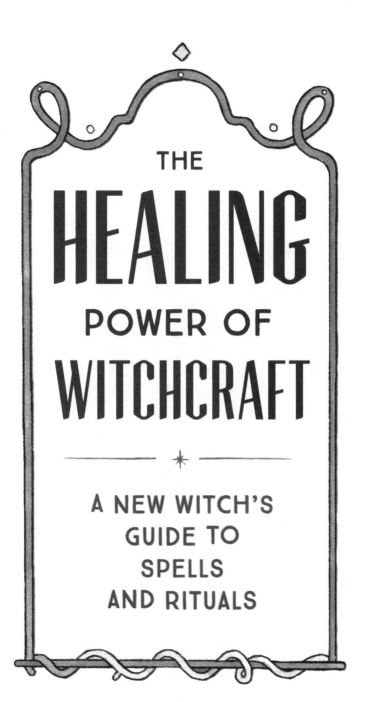

THE
HEALING
POWER OF
WITCHCRAFT

✦

A NEW WITCH'S
GUIDE TO
SPELLS
AND RITUALS

MEG ROSENBRIAR

ZEITGEIST • NEW YORK

Copyright © 2020 by Penguin Random House LLC

Published in the United States by Zeitgeist, an imprint of Zeitgeist™, a division of Penguin Random House LLC, New York.

penguinrandomhouse.com

Zeitgeist™ is a trademark of Penguin Random House LLC

ISBN: 9780593196809

Ebook ISBN: 9780593196816

Illustrations by Meredith Smallwood

Book design by Aimee Fleck

Printed in the United States of America

5 7 9 10 8 6 4

First Edition

✳

FOR THE KENTS

AND THE ROSYS

MAY YOU STAY

FOREVER YOUNG.

✳

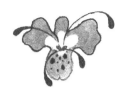
CONTENTS
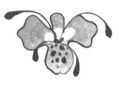

Merry Meet — 1

PART ONE WITCHCRAFT AND HEALING 4

1 Harnessing Your Power to Heal — 7

2 Preparing for Healing Work — 25

PART TWO HEAL YOURSELF 44

3 Heal Your Body — 46

4 Heal Your Mind — 78

5 Heal Your Spirit — 110

PART THREE HEAL YOUR COMMUNITY 144

6 Heal Your Friends and Family — 146

7 Heal Groups — 173

PART FOUR HEAL YOUR WORLD 204

8 Heal Your Home — 206

9 Heal the Planet — 235

10 Closing Thoughts — 266

Glossary — 267

Resources — 268

Index — 269

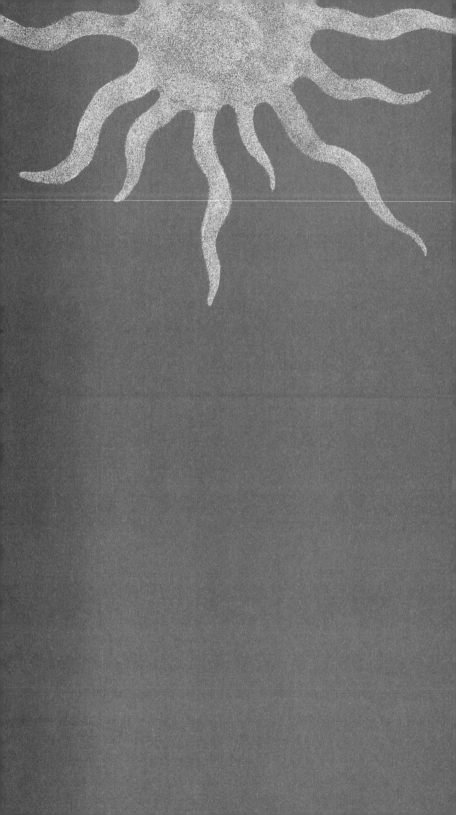

MERRY MEET

W‌elcome to the magickal world of healing through witchcraft. I am Meg, the Witch of the Shoreline, a witch devoted to healing through practical magick and intentional living. Although I hold both a bachelor's degree and a master's degree in religious studies, the most important learning and personal growth I have experienced has occurred at my witch altar. As a solitary practitioner, I began my witchcraft practice by connecting with myself and holding reverence for the cycles of nature. As I grew my inner witchy knowledge, a powerful thing happened. I actually grew my connectivity to my neighbors, communities, and my planet as well. I continue to find that the more witchy energy I engage in personally, the more witchy energy I can offer and share with others to help them and heal them.

I believe we all have the power to harness magick in order to heal ourselves, our communities, and our planet. Witches channel this power through intentional spellcraft, ritual, and contemplation. In Part 1, I will guide you toward your personal, merry path by familiarizing you with the elements of witchcraft you will need to know before beginning healing spellwork. In Parts 2, 3, and 4, I outline practical, healing magick you can perform for yourself, your communities, and your planet, respectively. While of course no one should replace or radically change their current health care plans without first talking to their doctor, this book serves as an alternative, holistic approach to wellness, guided by the fundamentals of witchcraft. It takes into account both bodily healing and emotional healing by addressing modern-day stresses with updated, modern witchcraft practices, created specifically for busy, contemporary witches.

This book is an accessible guide to healing witchcraft for even the newest of witches. It offers uncomplicated practices with which to explore your healing power. The spells provided within require only easy-to-find, inexpensive items. The magickal ingredients used are traditional plants, herbs, and spices designed to acquaint new witches with the basics of spellcraft. Nontraditional magickal ingredients, like crystals and essential oils, are also used to align your practice with modern wellness techniques that may already be working for you. Experienced witches will appreciate the comprehensive perspective and intuitive approach as a way to strengthen and expand their own established healing practices. All witches reading this book will discover just how powerful one witch can be at healing the world.

Witchcraft is as much about experiencing the journey as it is about reaching the destination. I wish you much peace and great success as you navigate your unique journey into healing witchcraft. So mote it be.

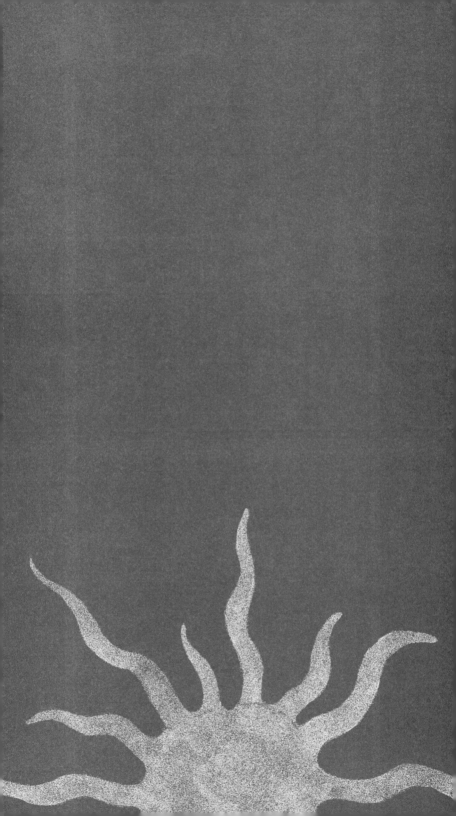

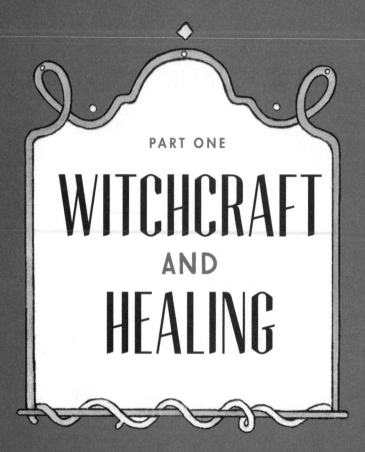

PART ONE

WITCHCRAFT

AND

HEALING

WITCHES CLAIM THEIR OWN BRAND OF MAGICK through awareness of their own being and awareness of the universal cycles of which they are a part. When the self or the self's environment is ailing or out of balance, witches know. Witches want to help, and they want to restore. As Ray Bradbury posited, "A Witch is born out of the true hungers of her time."

The good news is, all witches have an innate ability to perform healing magick. A witch may decide to follow a variety of paths in working witchcraft, but a wise witch knows working with magick that is abundant, healthy, and whole is the most powerful kind of magick. Thus, I believe all witches benefit from exploring magickal healing.

A witch understands their own intuition and their intent are the most powerful instruments they wield, but they allow magickal tools like herbs, oils, incantations, and timing to support their success. Working real magick for successful healing is certainly possible, but a witch first must become familiar with the elements and principles that support successful magick. This section of the book introduces you to everything you need to know before healing yourself, your communities, and the planet.

HARNESSING YOUR POWER TO HEAL

Witchcraft is the practice of magick. Magick is the harnessing of energy as a means to an end. Our universe is governed by interconnected energy and corresponding metaphysical properties. Witchcraft provides a conduit for these energies in order to create changes for the better. Healing witchcraft is the changing or dispersing of unwanted energy, with an aim of flourishing and achieving wholeness. As these old energies clear, and as new, healthy energies take root, the person or situation begins to heal. That, my witches, is what we mean by real magick.

The healing power of witchcraft comes from two sources—the witch and the universe. The witch is the agent, the creator. The universe provides the ingredients and recipe for our success. This chapter will guide you through the basics of witchcraft and provide you with the framework for the spells and rituals that follow. Let us begin by exploring seven tenets of witchcraft every witch should embrace in order to produce the most positive magickal results.

SEVEN GUIDING PRINCIPLES
OF WITCHCRAFT

———— ✳ ————

Witches commit themselves to guiding principles of the practice in order to create consistently powerful magick. Of course, the merry paths witches walk are as varied as witches themselves; nevertheless, these seven guiding principles provide the framework for magickal living.

1 CONNECTION TO SELF

Inscribed upon the entrance to the ancient temple of Delphi are two words: Know thyself. These words, survived through time immemorial, bear the same weight of wisdom today as they did for the ancients. You are your most powerful tool. It is your intuition, your wisdom, and your experience that powers all your magickal workings. As such, it is essential to get to know yourself. Once you uncover who you are, aside from who society tells you to be, and aside from traumatic experiences you have endured, you get down to the authentic, original witch. With a REAL witch, REAL magick happens.

How do you accomplish this process? Certainly not overnight! Remember to give yourself grace. Understand the process of delving within, often referred to as shadow work, can be messy and challenging. It is also incredibly empowering and a life-changing feat. In fact, I have found the more authentic the witch, the happier the witch.

Here are a few resources to get you started in connecting with yourself:

- Access an astrological birth chart calculator. There are many free calculators online and many books that will walk you through the meaning of your chart. Working through the placement of the planets at the time of your birth is incredibly revealing.

- Try other well-tested personality assessments like Myers–Briggs or Enneagram. See how they compare. What commonalities do you see? What areas are you proud of? What areas need work? Try taking these tests again throughout your lifetime to see if things have changed for you.

- Journaling, meditation, yoga, cooking, creating, and artistic pursuits are all excellent outlets for self-connection.

2 CONNECTION TO NATURE

Nature is our guide to the magickal world. Everything we need to make our will be done is contained in the vast web of energy that is our universe, including ourselves. Thus, getting to know the cycles and properties of our physical universe is essential to successful spellwork and healing. There are two parts to our universe—the heavens and the earth. We refer to the physical on Earth as nature and the heavens as the cosmos. Each has their own unique, but interconnected, cycles.

To connect with the cycle of earthly seasons, witchcraft celebrates eight sabbats or holidays, called the Wheel of the Year. Beginning with Samhain (Halloween) as Witches' New Year, the Wheel of the Year follows along with the change in seasons, marking beginnings and endings as we journey through each year. Here is a brief chart of the eight sabbats, the date they usually fall on, and the season they herald. I have

SABBAT	DATE	MARKING
SAMHAIN	October 31	Witches' New Year
YULE (WINTER SOLSTICE)	December 21	Start of winter
IMBOLC	February 1	Midpoint between winter and spring
OSTARA (VERNAL EQUINOX)	March 20	Start of spring
BELTANE	May 1	Midpoint between spring and summer
LITHA (SUMMER SOLSTICE)	June 21	Start of summer
LAMMAS	August 1	Midpoint between summer and autumn
MABON (AUTUMNAL EQUINOX)	September 23	Start of autumn

FOCUS	COLOR THEME	SYMBOLS
Third harvest, endings, communing with the spirit world	Orange, black, purple	Pumpkins, leaves, acorn, veil
Rebirth	Red, green, silver, gold, white	Evergreen, pine cone, holly, yule logs
First fertility festival, hope	Green, white, red	Candles, flame, cauldron, snowdrops
Second fertility festival, beginnings	Green, yellow, pink, white, lavender	Eggs, newborn animals, plant sprouts
Third fertility festival, sexuality	Green, bright colors	Florals, greenery
Duality, balance	Green, yellow, gold, red	Sunflowers, bees, butterflies
First harvest, security	Yellow, brown, gold	Bread loaf, corn dollies
Second harvest, abundance	Gold, orange, brown, red, dark green	Fruits, nuts, grains

noted corresponding themes, colors, and symbols you may use as décor on your altar/in your home to streamline the energy of each sabbat into your surroundings. Note that exact dates may vary slightly year to year since the astronomy each sabbat is based upon varies slightly each year. By marking these key dates of our year, witches are able to process change by shedding the old and embracing the new.

3 CONNECTION TO THE COSMOS

A witch understands they have a place in the universe. A witch is not simply a free-floating form but a being deeply connected to the cycles of our celestial bodies. The sun and moon affect the witch, their powers, and their work. By living intentionally, alongside these cycles, a witch aligns themselves with success in spellwork and healing. Yes, one can absolutely perform a spell and not adhere to the guidelines offered to us by the cosmos. Nothing bad will come of it. However, it is far wiser to align your spells with cosmic energy, as it gives an instant power boost to your craft. A quick consultation of where the sun and moon are placed allows you to tailor the most effective spell method for that timing.

THE SUN

You are probably familiar with the Western zodiac. It begins in the sign of Aries on the spring equinox in March. As Earth orbits the sun, the sun appears to progress through the zodiac chart according to the schedule on the next page. Each zodiac contains its own unique energy flow, and each zodiac sign is rooted in a particular corresponding element: fire, earth, air, or water.

SIGN	DATES	ELEMENT
ARIES	March 21– April 19	Fire
TAURUS	April 20– May 20	Earth
GEMINI	May 21– June 20	Air
CANCER	June 21– July 22	Water
LEO	July 23– August 22	Fire
VIRGO	August 23– September 22	Earth
LIBRA	September 23– October 22	Air
SCORPIO	October 23– November 21	Water
SAGITTARIUS	November 22– December 21	Fire
CAPRICORN	December 22– January 19	Earth
AQUARIUS	January 20– February 18	Air
PISCES	February 19– March 20	Water

THE MOON

The moon cycles through the zodiac in the same order as the sun, changing zodiac locations roughly every two and a half days instead of every month like the sun. Note: Brief periods when the moon is not in any zodiac sign are referred to as "void of course." These periods are generally regarded as time to rest and not perform magick, as energy is chaotic and vapid during this time.

The phase of the moon impacts magickal workings as well. Listed below are corresponding spell types to moon phases. For the purposes of this book, we will focus mainly on the timing of the new moon and the full moon, but many of the spells may be done in the two-week waning and waxing periods as well. Remember, you do not have to wait for the moon to be in the suggested phase to perform a spell. You may also use any phase of the moon to charge magickal materials. The moon is intrinsic to witchcraft at any phase. Besides, the bulk of the magick is in your intention; aligning with the appropriate moon phase simply helps the spell along to success.

NEW MOON: Best for spells for fresh starts, new relationships, new business ventures, new knowledge or awareness, letting go of the past

WAXING CRESCENT: Best for spells for family, learning, growth, goal manifestation, path revelation

FIRST QUARTER: Best for spells for strength, durability, stamina, goals, and achievement

WAXING GIBBOUS: Best for spells for money, abundance, competence, positive changes, and robust health

FULL MOON: Best for spells for healing, intuition, and witchy power

WANING GIBBOUS: Best for spells involving breaking bad habits and ending toxic relationships

LAST QUARTER: Best for spells for restorative healing, patching strained relationships, kitchen and hearth witchery

WANING CRESCENT: Best for spells of restful healing, self-love, and banishing

4 COMMITMENT TO KNOWLEDGE AND LEARNING

The goal of a witch is constant self-growth and transformation. Some witches are slow and steady learners, preferring to stick to what they know but enriching their practice with deliberate, curated ideas. Other witches voraciously move from one subject to another, learning all they can. Perhaps you fall somewhere in the middle. The point is, static has no place in witchcraft. As the outer world evolves and grows, so must the witch in order to maintain balance and clarity. The reward, of course, is wisdom—a virtue only to be extolled through praxis.

5 SALUBRIOUS, INTENTIONAL LIVING

Our bodies are the vessels that support our magick-making. Taking care of our body through salubrious, healthful living is a top priority to ensure output is as powerful as possible. This is not to say witches don't spend some weekends eating junk food and watching every single Harry Potter movie.

However, the overall goal of the witch is to make wellness choices that benefit their physical health. Choosing to eat healthy, stretch, exercise, and enjoy treats in moderation all contribute to boosting power in spellwork.

A witch also uses their intention to aid in their mental health. Living in the moment, or intentional living, is much more than focusing on the positives. Yes, that mindset is extremely important and powerful, but intentional living is really about acceptance and release. Instead of engaging anxiety about the future, or regret about the past, live your best life in the moment you are in. It is the best use of your energy to focus on what you can accomplish at the moment. Of course, restoration is also an intentional, essential part of a witchy path, so don't forget to make resting part of your daily routine as well.

6 JOYFUL, CELEBRATORY LIVING

A witch understands the magickal value in celebrating life's moments. This is not to say a witch is blind to sorrow or pain—quite the opposite, actually. A witch celebrates life's achievements, milestones, and beauty because of the sorrow and the pain within and without. If we are to feel deeply, connect broadly, and restore wholly, then a joyful approach to living, despite the odds, is a truly magickal thing indeed.

Perhaps your commute to work is hellish, but the sunrise in the distance is truly something to admire. No, the sunrise might not make up for some awful drivers, but it is not supposed to. The steadfast sun is there in commiseration, companionship, and inspiration. "See, witch?" says the sun. "I will keep rising, and you will keep enjoying it." Moments like that show you how joyful, celebratory living softens your edges and invites magickal, healing vibes into your life.

7 FOLLOW THE DUALISTIC ENERGY CODE

Finally, every witch is mindful of this ancient universal energy code, attributed to Hermes Trismegistus, the father of hermeticism:

As above so below
As within so without
As the universe
So the soul

For every action, there is a reaction. For every macrocosm, there is a microcosm. For every soul, there is a star. Witches strive to honor and keep space for this balance to flourish and grow. It is the ordered way, and witches embrace this dualistic reality in order to align themselves and their magick with energy's great power.

YOUR PATH TO WITCHCRAFT

Everyone has their own unique path to witchcraft. Aside from the few who are born into witchy families, most witches begin practicing witchcraft later in life. However, out of those who begin practicing later in life, the majority describe common callings or feelings that they were destined for a witchcrafted life all along. Some signs you are called to witchcraft include the following:

- You feel a special relationship with the moon and stars, often staring at them longingly and in companionship.

- Animals are drawn to you, ladybugs and butterflies land on you, strays find you.

- You feel deeply connected to the cycles of the seasons, nature, and plants.

- You are called to collect shells, rocks, bones, crystals, and other gifts from the earth.

- You are an empath or highly sensitive person.

- You are calmed by water, either by submerging yourself in it or simply being near it.

- You notice repeating number patterns and other seemingly coincidental patterns.

- You have a strong sense of intuition or knowing.

- Contemporary, patriarchal-based religions no longer resonate with you.

- You seek community based on commonality, not hierarchy.

- You feel compelled to help and heal others.

WHAT TYPE OF WITCH ARE YOU?

Any internet search will reveal several hundred lists of different types of witches. Identity is clearly important. I have provided a brief reference list below of common witch "types" to give you a solid introduction as you formulate your own witchy path.

ELEMENTAL WITCH: Works with one or a combination of the elements (earth, air, water, fire) in their practice

COSMIC WITCH: Works with astrology, the cycles of the sun and moon, birth charts

GLAMOUR WITCH: Works with love, beauty, self-love, and enchantment spells

HEDGE WITCH: A solitary healer, working with herbs and plants, engaging in divination and liminal work

GREEN WITCH: A caretaker of plants, nature, and gardens, and creates natural wellness tinctures

KITCHEN WITCH: Cooks with magickal ingredients and magickal intention

HEARTH WITCH: Homemakers with magickal intention

ECLECTIC WITCH: A modern term used to describe a witch with many different pursuits

This list is certainly not exhaustive, and many witches dabble in different types of witchcraft, as evidenced by the final term, eclectic witch. In fact, this book intentionally draws on all of these types of witches. This is because all types of witches are healers. Witches aim to walk a more connected, healthier approach to whatever path matters to them, be it crystal magick, love magick, manifestation magick, spiritual coaching, herbal magick, or something else entirely. This book is essential for all types of witches as they engage in their chosen path.

SOLITARY WITCH OR COVEN?

A solitary witch traditionally practices witchcraft alone, while a coven is a group of witches who practice witchcraft together.

 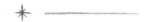

Each witch may decide for themselves which form of practice they prefer. However, in this age of information, even the witch who prefers to practice alone is most likely influenced by social media and current trends in witchcraft. Likewise, the witch who practices as part of a coven still has access to witchcraft materials extending far beyond the coven in the form of the great grimoire, Google. The sheer accessibility modernity has given witchcraft makes for a new, more flexible dichotomy between the solitary practitioner and the coven.

My suggestion to the fledgling witch is to set aside this dichotomy and focus on finding like-minded individuals to grow the knowledge with. The advent of social media has made finding witchy friends a real possibility in a way witchcraft has never experienced. Explore hashtags on Instagram that call to you, such as #crystals or #firewitch, and see what people using that hashtag are saying. Join the conversation and meet colleagues. As we adjust antiquated modes of thinking about community, especially the coven, we adjust the individual's freedom to seek the most effective methods for their practice. Find your people and get to know them. Join forces from there if you feel it is right for your practice.

A WITCH'S STATE OF MIND

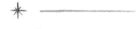

For spellwork to be most effective, the practitioner needs to be in a calm, open, and positive mental state. Our emotions are energetically charged, and when we are not in control of them, the energy of our magickal workings is influenced unduly. Before practicing craft, take time to slow yourself down with some deep breaths or centering methods. Meditation in particular allows us to practice guiding our will and holding space for peace. Since witchcraft is all about willfully directing energy, your state of mind matters greatly.

SETTING CLEAR, POWERFUL INTENTIONS

Once you are centered and ready to craft, the first step is to set clear, powerful intentions for your spellwork. You want to work out exactly what it is you would like the spell to accomplish. This helps the universe understand the type of energy you are trying to conjure. It also allows you to be clear with yourself about your hopes and expectations. An example of a clear, powerful intention would be, "I am working this healing spell to ease my anxiety so I can sleep better tonight." This type of articulation is much more powerful than simply thinking, "Gee, I hope this anti-anxiety spell does something." Watch your power blossom exponentially once you start honing your intentions.

THE WELL-APPOINTED ALTAR

One of the best ways to hone your intentions for spellcraft is to reflect them in your altar setup. Altars are as unique and varied as the witches who build them, but all altars have key components for successful spellwork.

LOCATION

Choose a location that is both practical and meaningful. Make sure whatever area you choose to devote to altar space is out of the way of major household traffic and safe from curious hands. This is also sacred space, so choose an area that empowers you. Select a cozy corner of your bedroom, or a special table near your fireplace, or a space with a great window—wherever you feel most inspired.

SURFACE

Altars are often beautiful, but first and foremost they are a workspace. Allow enough space to accomplish any work you may need to do, like grinding herbs, pulling tarot cards, or creating a crystal grid.

THE FOUR ELEMENTS

A witch uses the four elements to power their spellwork. As such, altars should have symbols that pay homage to them. Here are some commonly used items to represent the elements:

AIR: Wand, feather, bells, books, incense

FIRE: Candle, athame, phallus, pyramid, ash

WATER: Chalice, bowl, crystal ball, moonwater, seashell

EARTH: Pentacle, coin, stone, plant, flower, bone, seeds

A candle is one of the handiest tools in witchcraft because it represents all four elements. The flame is fire, the candle wick and body are earth, the melting wax is water, and the smoke is air.

CORRESPONDENCES

While not necessary, it is a useful practice to add correspondences to your altar. This means you dress your altar with items that represent, or correspond, to your spellwork goals.

For example, when performing a spell for self-love, placing a rose quartz crystal on your altar helps amplify the spell's power because rose quartz is a stone associated with self-love. You will find the act of researching suitable altar correspondences to support your spellwork really starts to grow your knowledge of the different energies of witchcraft.

SELECTING YOUR WITCH MODE

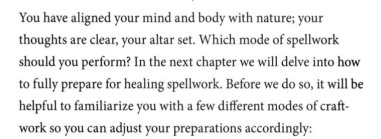

You have aligned your mind and body with nature; your thoughts are clear, your altar set. Which mode of spellwork should you perform? In the next chapter we will delve into how to fully prepare for healing spellwork. Before we do so, it will be helpful to familiarize you with a few different modes of craftwork so you can adjust your preparations accordingly:

RITUALS: A ritual is a premeditated set of magickal steps honoring or inviting a chosen energy. Rituals are meant to align, cleanse, and enhance rather than change or transform.

CHARMS: Charms are objects, or a gathering of objects, that correspond to drawing a certain energy. Charms attract the energy of their contents.

SPELL CASTING: A spell is an ordered, intentional manipulation of natural energy as a means to an end.

POTIONS: Potions are concoctions intentionally crafted with magickal ingredients to bring about change.

INDIVIDUAL MAGICK VERSUS SYMPATHY MAGICK

In Part 2, you will find spells to heal your body, mind, and spirit and will use individual magick to do so since the focus is on yourself. Parts 3 and 4 are full of spells to help your community, friends, family, groups, and planet. You are performing the magick on their behalf; thus it is called sympathy magick. Rest assured, a self-healed witch has all the tools they need to help others in their healing process; sympathy magick will guide you in working spells for others.

STEPPING INTO YOUR POWER

This chapter provided you with the foundations of successful witchcraft, especially witchcraft for healing purposes. As you digest this information, keep in mind that the journey of witchcraft is a long and winding process. No one can expect to be proficient overnight, let alone an expert. It is also worthwhile to keep in mind that all the study in the world cannot replace the lived experience of stepping up and actually practicing some witchcraft. Are you ready to begin, my witches?

PREPARING FOR HEALING WORK

Preparing your space and yourself for healing is a vital part of witchcraft. Think of preparing as an act of intention setting. By selecting your methods and tools and organizing them, the mind processes the properties of the spell and begins to channel the energies needed for successful spellwork. In the last chapter, we learned the basic tenets of witchcraft. This chapter focuses on how to prepare both practically and spiritually for healing work using our foundational knowledge of witchcraft.

In the pages that follow, I will walk you through the basics of common magickal healing tools and ingredients, including herbs, spices, crystals, and essential oils. I will also offer witchy methods like grounding and energy raising with which to achieve optimum spell power. Once you are familiar with the tools and methods of the craft, it will be time to cast some healing spells.

THE WITCH'S CUPBOARD

※

As you journey down your healing path, you will undoubtedly collect many magickal ingredients and meaningful items to aid you with your craft. For the purposes of this book, I have selected 10 herbs, 10 spices, 10 crystals, and 10 essential oils to get you started. These magickal ingredients are selected specifically as easy-to-use, easily found or purchased, and common in spellwork. Additionally, common household items aid in the practice of spellwork. Let us rummage through the witch's cupboard now, beginning with the essentials every witch needs to get started.

THE ESSENTIALS

Begin by securing the essential tools of successful witchcraft. There are seven tools every witch should have in their cupboard:

WHITE CANDLES: The candle is a universal magickal tool, as it represents all four elements. White is the universal magickal color. A white candle can take the place of any color candle in a spell. For simplicity's sake, all candle use in this book will be with a white candle. I recommend securing chime-size candles, as they are small, easy to work with, and burn quickly.

SALT: Salt absorbs negative energy, grounds, delineates, and protects. For this book I use basic white table salt unless otherwise noted.

ROSEMARY (HERB AND OIL): Similar to white candles, rosemary is the universal witch's herb. Use it in place of any other herb or oil in spellwork.

CLEAR QUARTZ CRYSTAL: As with rosemary and white candles, clear quartz is the universal crystal. Use it in place of other crystals should you not have them in your repertoire.

CAULDRON: You need a safe vessel in which to perform fire magick and to hold hot water for various rituals and spells. If you do not have a cauldron, a heat-safe bowl should work just fine.

ATHAME: An athame, or ritual knife, comes in handy for consecrating, cutting, and engraving magickal tools. The athame also represents the element of fire on an altar, which is particularly handy when open flame or smoke is not feasible.

JARS AND CONTAINERS: A by-product of proper witching is certainly the multitude of magickal ingredients one starts to collect. Save those empty pickle jars and coffee tins, and definitely find some mason jars to organize your magickal wares.

HERBS

Herbalism is one of the most effective healing methods available, as evidenced by thousands of years of use and study by our healer ancestors. Individual plants have properties that can be used medically, depending on how they are prepared and applied. Did you know these same plants have metaphysical healing properties as well? Consider the interconnectedness of nature and our elemental wholeness. Just as a plant has physical properties we can identify, like leaf shape, aroma, growing patterns, and medicinal uses, so does each plant have magickal healing properties we harness for healing witchcraft.

The 10 introductory herbs listed below are common and can be found at most food markets and gardening centers. You can buy these herbs dried or in live plant form. If you are just starting out, I recommend securing all herbs listed in dried form so you have them readily at your disposal, and then branching out into plant cultivation from there. Alternatively, most grocery stores have fresh-cut herb leaves in their produce section, often located by the bagged salads. This is a great way to obtain fresh herbs and sprigs when the spell requires them without needing the whole plant. You can even buy them when you don't need them and dry them for when you do. Be sure to store your dried herbs in a cool, dry, shaded location to keep their integrity.

Regardless of how you get your magickal hands on these herbs, when you receive your herbs, be sure to say hello! Thank them for their magick. Tell them you infuse them with your love and your will. Build a relationship with your magickal helpers before using them to encourage energy connectivity.

The herbs I have selected are all healing helpers that either promote health or help attract healing energy. I have also listed the additional magickal properties of each herb to give you a sense of the type of healing energy they lend themselves to.

BASIL (*OCIMUM BASILICUM*): Love, happiness, abundance, tranquility

OREGANO (*ORIGANUM VULGARE*): Peace, grounding, release, balance

PARSLEY (*PETROSELINUM CRISPUM*): Protection, spiritual connection, vitality, passion

LAVENDER (*LAVANDULA ANGUSTIFOLIA*): Calming, sleep aid, uplifting, spiritual connection

THYME (*THYMUS VULGARIS*): Purification, strength, bravery, love, attraction

CHAMOMILE (*CHAMAEMELUM NOBILE*): Cleansing, soothes anxiety, balance

SAGE (*SALVIA OFFICINALIS*): Longevity, cleansing, protection, psychic powers

ROSEMARY (*ROSMARINUS OFFICINALIS*): Cleansing, fidelity, longevity, wisdom, memory

MINT (*MENTHA*): Abundance, success, prosperity, joy, fertility, renewal

BAY LEAF (*LAURUS NOBILIS*): Divination, wish granting, protection, purification, strength

SPICES

Herbs are the leaf of the plant while spices are made up of all other parts of the plant, including seeds, flowers, berries, bark, and roots. For our magickal healing purposes, I have chosen common spices you may already own, use in your cooking, or add to your smoothies or shakes to give yourself a boost. The more familiar you are with your ingredients, the more effective the spellwork. As such, spices are a great addition to the cupboard of the beginner witch. Like herbs, store them in a shaded, cool, dry location.

We will use these spices in our healing spellwork. They all have magickal healing properties. Their additional magickal properties are listed as well to help you associate the type of healing energy each spice provides.

ALLSPICE (*PIMENTA OFFICINALIS*): Love, luck, prosperity, abundance

TURMERIC (*CURCUMA LONGA*): Purification, grounding

BLACK PEPPER (*PIPER NIGRUM*): Courage, banish negativity, protection

ANISE (*PIMPINELLA ANISUM*): Psychic awareness, good luck, prosperity, calming

CAYENNE (*CAPSICUM ANNUUM*): Accelerates, separates, cleanses, repels negativity

NUTMEG (*MYRISTICA FRAGRANS*): Prosperity, luck, abundance, connection, breaking cycles

CLOVE (*SYZYGIUM AROMATICUM*): Protection, divination, stress relief, prosperity, relationship

CINNAMON (*CINNAMOMUM VERUM*): Success, wealth, love, lust, grounding

GARLIC (*ALLIUM SATIVUM*): Protection, invigorating, passion

GINGER (*ZINGIBER OFFICINALE*): Energy, abundance, balance, sexuality

CRYSTALS

Crystals are the adornment of Mother Earth, beautiful gifts from our planet meant to be used in magick. Crystals act as natural batteries, transferring their innate high-energy vibrations to lower-vibrating energy sources like humans. Their energy can be attuned to our magickal purposes, particularly for healing.

You can find the crystals below at any local crystal and gem shop or online. Just one small crystal is enough to make a noticeable difference in energy, so do not feel the need to rush to purchase anything huge or expensive. It is preferable to purchase stones in person, always from reputably mined sources, as it allows you to feel their energy up front. However, since this is not always possible, it is always a good idea to purify and charge your crystals to yourself once you bring them home. Spend time with your new crystals. Imprint your energy on them and theirs onto you. Get to know their unique energy, as some crystals absorb negative energy and some crystals amplify positive energy. All crystals transform energy for the benefit of magickal healing.

The energy of crystals dulls as they are handled or used, much like a battery. Here are five easy ways to both welcome new crystals and recharge your existing crystals:

1. Place them outside under moonlight and leave them overnight.

2. Wrap them in a towel with a clear quartz crystal and leave together for 24 hours.

3. Bury them in dirt for a few days.

4. Pass them through smoke.

5. Bathe them in sound, from a bell, gong, or drum.

NOTE: Avoid immersing crystals in water for any length of time unless you are sure they are water-friendly crystals. Wipe down crystals with a cloth to physically clean them.

Here are the crystals we will rely on for our spells and their energy properties:

BLACK TOURMALINE (ABSORBING): Strength and confidence

CITRINE (AMPLIFYING): Willpower, confidence, self-expression, creativity

ROSE QUARTZ (AMPLIFYING): Love and self-care

SODALITE (AMPLIFYING): Peace, balance, and harmony

SMOKY QUARTZ (AMPLIFYING): Rest, renewal

GREEN AVENTURINE (AMPLIFYING): Courage, abundance, steadfastness, loyalty

JASPER (ABSORBING): Grounding, calming

FLUORITE (ABSORBING): Cleansing, synthesizes negative energy, clarity

CARNELIAN (ABSORBING): Creativity, inspiration, passion

AMETHYST (AMPLIFYING): Wisdom, knowledge, harmony, balance

ESSENTIAL OILS

Essential oils are compounds of plants extracted for their aroma, helping properties, and yes, magick. These oils are easily obtained online, in pharmacies, at many major retailers, and even in some grocery stores. Look for them near the candle section of the store.

Since these are pungent, powerful oils, we often want ways to diffuse them or use them more subtly than through direct contact. Thus, when using essential oils, you want to obtain both a diffuser and a carrier oil or two to help you work with them. For our purposes, a mini/personal diffuser is absolutely acceptable and can be purchased for under $20. Carrier oil is an unscented oil that helps dilute and transport the essential oils for specific uses like face masks, creams, and potions. The carrier oil you choose is purely personal preference. I prefer olive or grapeseed oil for stovetop use, jojoba oil for aromatherapy use, and coconut oil for topical salves.

The really good news is that all essential oils contain healing magick. Since they are derived from the very natural essence of the plants, trees, flowers, herbs, and spices used in witchery, they are concentrated, powerful healing helpers and an important addition to the cupboard of the modern witch. Below are the oils we will use in this book and their magickal correspondences.

BASIL: Romance, affection, luck, inspiration, connection

SWEET ORANGE: Confidence, joy, abundance, friendship, good cheer

FRANKINCENSE: Spirituality, purifying, cleansing, intuition, connection

BERGAMOT: Mood lifter, confidence, clarity

YLANG-YLANG: Euphoric, sensual, passionate, lustful

CEDAR: Stability, grounding, strength

PEPPERMINT: Concentration, focus, centering, performance enhancing

LAVENDER: Calming, soothing, intuitive

EUCALYPTUS: Invigorating, relieves exhaustion, enhances creativity

TEA TREE: Cleansing, purifying, pain relieving

ADDITIONAL TOOLS

Here are additional tools to aid you in your spellwork. These are not necessary, as they all can easily be replaced with other tools or methods, but having them can make the spellcraft process easier.

BELL: Bells represent the element of air and are excellent tools for clearing negative energy or releasing energy during spellwork.

MORTAR AND PESTLE: Use this tool to grind up herbs into fine powders.

COMMON HOUSEHOLD ITEMS: Witchcraft relies on the mundane as much as the magickal, as is fitting of a method that creates real change. Feel empowered to get creative with your household tools. For example, if a spell calls for twine, perhaps you use leftover giftwrapping ribbon. The practical function of the object is more important than the objects themselves in this case. Here are some of the common household items used in this book: string, twine, ribbon, cloth, scissors, small muslin bags, cheesecloth, apples, oranges, lemons, honey, sugar, lighter, bowls of varying sizes, cooking pots, teacups, cotton balls, and towels.

METHODS USED IN SPELLCRAFT

This book relies on a few different methods used in spellcraft, which are worth reviewing for new witches.

ANOINTING

Anointing is the process of applying oil to a candle or another tool in order to magickally charge it. How much oil you use in the anointing process is purely personal preference, and even just one drop of oil will do the trick. The magick lies in the intention of the application.

DRESSING A CANDLE

Dressing a candle refers to the process of adding herbs for magickal purposes to the outside of the candle after anointing the candle. If the spell calls for dressing a candle, I recommend using several drops of oil to ensure the candle is fully oiled. You will roll your oiled candle in the herbs before you light it, and the herbs will stick to the candle as an added magickal correspondence to your healing workings.

ASPERGING

Asperging is the process of sprinkling objects with magickally charged water to transfer the magickal properties onto the object. This books uses fresh herbs to dip into your magickal water and shake, or asperge, onto other objects during healing work.

SYMBOLS FOR THE ELEMENTS

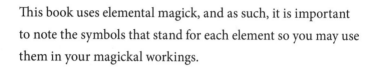

This book uses elemental magick, and as such, it is important to note the symbols that stand for each element so you may use them in your magickal workings.

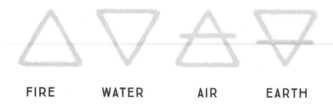

FIRE   WATER   AIR   EARTH

Additionally, in our workings to heal our planet, we will use this symbol to stand for Earth. Note that this symbol and connotation are deliberately different from earth the element.

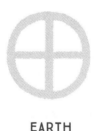

EARTH

SETTING THE STAGE FOR HEALING WORK

---- ✳ ----

The moment to cast a spell for healing has come. You are ready, witch. Time to fully step into your power, armed with knowledge and helpful tools to heal yourself, your neighborhoods, and your world. These following final steps guide you through the process of preparing to cast a spell.

ALIGNING YOUR SPELL TIMING

When it comes to choosing the perfect time to cast a spell, there are a number of energy cycles you may consult, but nothing is more important than following your intuition. If you feel called to move certain energies immediately, do so. There is no need to wait until the perfect time according to standard witchery when you, the witch, are ready and moved to cast.

MOON PHASE

The most common way to select the optimum timing for any given spell is by following the cycles of the moon. In Chapter 1, we covered the corresponding moon phases and spellwork, so refer to that chart as guidance on moon cycle spell casting. The phases of the moon represent the natural cycle of energy you will note in the "Suggested timing" section of certain spells. Again, you may perform a spell at any time that feels right to you, and nothing bad will come of going against the moon cycle. The spell simply may not be as effective.

THE MAGICKAL TOOL OF GROUNDING

Grounding is the process of connecting your mind and body to the energy needed for spellwork. A number of tasks can help you ground yourself, including readying your work space and yourself.

Selecting the space in which to perform your witchcraft and preparing that space are integral parts of successful spellwork. Many witches have a dedicated indoor altar, but at the very least make sure you have a quiet, comfortable area of your home to engage in spiritual workings. The space should be tidy and organized. You don't want anything distracting your energy. Furthermore, it is a good idea to identify a dedicated outdoor location where you may perform spellwork in privacy. Many workings require direct connection with nature, and invoking Mother Earth is powerful indeed. Either way, before performing spellwork in your dedicated sacred space, be sure to burn some purifying herbs like bay leaf or sage to reset the area's energy and ground your intentions.

Casting a circle is a common and effective way to define your space for magickal workings. It also affords protection and amplifies the energies conjured during spellwork. While not necessary for most beginner spellwork, casting a circle is an important part of witchcraft for many witches, as they use it to embrace the liminality of magickal workings. Begin by physically defining your circle with salt or crystals. More experienced witches may define their circles with just their own energy, which is certainly fine, but a clear marking is helpful for beginner witches.

There are many ways to cast a circle, but one of the most effective is calling corners. Sometimes called calling quarters, the name refers to the invocation of the four directions and their corresponding elements. Once your space is purified and your circle drawn, ring your altar bell three times (or tap a pot with a spoon if you don't have a bell) and speak the following incantation:

Face north and raise your arms. Say:

"Northern earth, I call you to my aid."

Lower arms and turn east. Raise arms and say:

"Eastern air, I call you to my aid."

Lower arms and turn south. Raise arms and say:

"Southern fire, I call you to my aid."

Lower arms and turn west. Raise arms and say:

"Western water, I call you to my aid."

Lower your arms, center yourself on your altar, and incant:

"I thank the elements on this hour
For casting this circle in healing power."

SETTING INTENTIONS

As discussed in Chapter 1, intention setting is the cornerstone of spellwork. All the tools in the world are no replacement for your own willpower. After all, you are the witch. The herbs, oils, and crystals help the witch, but it is you who actually makes the magick. Speak your intention aloud just before you begin to raise your energy level for spell casting. Clearly articulating your goal for the spell will keep your energies on track, channeled, and most effective.

RAISING ENERGY

Raising energy is the last step in preparation for spellwork. This is the moment you begin to engage with energy to harness it for healing, just before you start your spellwork. Quite simply, any method that tunes you in to energy and aligns you with its power is effective. Here are a few ways to raise energy. Pay attention to what you feel as you try them. Hone your tactics until you have the perfect ritual for yourself:

BALL OF ENERGY METHOD: Stand firmly in your sacred space. Press your palms together in prayer fashion and rub them together vigorously. You will immediately start to feel friction and warmth. That is energy! Sink into the flow. See if you can form a ball of energy between your hands. Imagine it as a glowing bulb you can expand around your entire altar to power your workings.

ENJOY YOURSELF: Happy witches are powerful witches. Put on music you love. Dance and sing. Move your body rhythmically. Masturbation or sex with a partner are other options to raise energy. Some witches enjoy a glass of wine to help free the ego and let the soul do its thing.

MEDITATION: Some witches feel more powerful sitting still and drawing energy to them via meditation. This is also an extremely powerful method and a bit more advanced, as the practitioner should be familiar with the powers of meditation before applying them to witchcraft for the most effective energy raising.

CLOSING THE CIRCLE

Proceed with your spellwork. When finished, ring the bell again three times and then recite:

"Now the bell has been rung. Let this circle be undone."

The energy is released and your spell is complete.

REBALANCING ENERGY

After spellwork, it is common to feel exhausted or foggy. Some witches even report period-like symptoms. Take care of yourself. You just moved entire fields of energy! Of course you are going to feel depleted. This doesn't mean you are weak or ill equipped for spellwork. It simply means you are on the waning cycle of your power and must rest until you feel ready to begin again. This tiredness is entirely natural and something to embrace. Like any muscle, the more magick you perform over time, the more strength and endurance you will have.

Here are a few ways to rebalance energy after spellwork:

- Drink chamomile tea

- Stretch and/or meditate

- Journal about your spellwork experience

- Practice earthing: walk barefoot outside and soak in the balance of the natural earth through your feet

- Bathe in Epsom salt, peppermint oil, and sweet orange oil

Take care of yourself, dear witch. We need you to help with the important task of healing ourselves, our communities, and our world.

SPELLWORK CLEANUP

In the spells that follow, I offer suggestions, when appropriate, on how to clean up and dispose of leftover magickal materials. These materials may have negative energies transferred to them, or the disposal may even be part of the spell. In general, try to return used organic spell matter to the earth by burying or scattering the leftovers outdoors. At the very least, bring all spellwork leftovers to a bin outside your home to release the energy from your space. Additionally, it is extremely important to ensure that no candles are left burning or unattended at any point. Be sure candles are fully snuffed out once your spellwork is finished by dipping the wick in some water or using a snuffer. Cleanup releases us from the energies we raised and is a necessary step to complete spellwork.

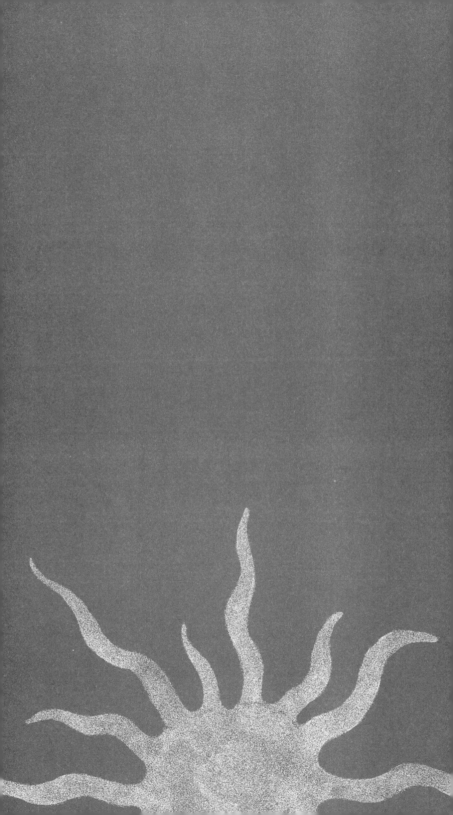

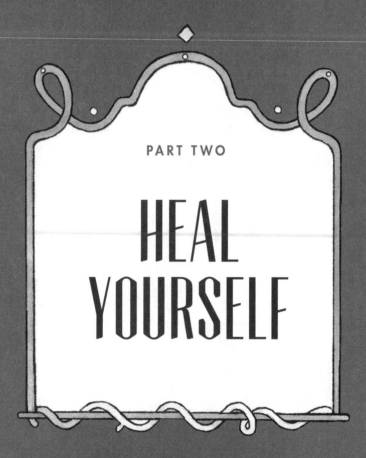

PART TWO

HEAL YOURSELF

BEFORE YOU CAN HEAL OTHERS OR THE WORLD, you will need to heal yourself. Addressing your personal health gives you the building blocks you will need to command successful healing when working at large. The self may be healed in three ways: body, mind, and spirit. The healed body supports the energy needed for spellwork. The healed mind allows for clarity and intention to flow freely. The healed spirit readies you to share your healing light with your community and the world.

Remember, healing is an ongoing process and is often not linear. It is an act of self-kindness to release any expectations you have about the healing process. Allow yourself the grace you need to try to heal, and the rest will follow as you engage in the work of healing. You will find meaning through this work; in fact, healing is about the courage to return to sources of pain and address them as needed. Witchcraft offers actionable methods with which to heal, and it is my honor to share them with you.

Here are rituals and spells for healing your body, mind, and spirit. My hope is that you may return to them again and again, as needed, with fresh perspective, to ever strengthen your healing powers.

3

HEAL YOUR BODY

Your body is the vessel for your willpower and magick abilities. Helping your body become and stay as healthy as possible is a worthy goal in order to engage quality magickal output. Applying witchcraft to bodily healing work means utilizing magickal healing tools in the form of spells and rituals to create healing energy for the body. It is helpful to think of magickal bodily healing as an alignment of the body with the natural rhythms of elements that have healing properties. By tuning in to your magickal ingredients with your senses and your actions in the physical realm, the body begins to heal using the metaphysical energy produced. Let us now turn to the magickal act of healing your body.

GOOD MORNING, SUNSHINE

PURPOSE OF SPELL: Charge your crystals, and your **body**, with energy for the day by calling on the four directions in a **magickal** blessing.

SUGGESTED TIMING:
Just after awakening for the day

ITEMS NEEDED:
- Candle
- Lighter

MAGICKAL INGREDIENTS:
- 1 tablespoon dried thyme **or a** few sprigs of fresh **thyme**
- 1 citrine crystal
- 1 carnelian crystal
- 3 drops orange oil

SPELLWORK

✦ Nestle your crystals on a bed of thyme. As you do, **release** yourself from wanting to go back to bed and transfer **that** energy to the neatly placed crystals. Allow them to soak **in the** energy of strength from the bed of thyme.

✦ Anoint your candle with the oil. At the same time, **notice your** body beginning to ready and cleanse itself for the day **ahead.** Send these vibes of optimism into your oil and candle **with your** fingers by rubbing in a deosil, or clockwise, motion. Wash **your** hands free of the oil. Light your candle of energetic joy.

CONTINUED >>>

✦ Pick up each crystal, one in each hand, and make a fist around each one. Feel the energizing properties of the thyme-charged citrine and carnelian race up your arms and into your body. Imagine the energy swirling around your insides, bringing you renewal.

✦ Face east. Thrust your hands straight out in front of you, opening your fingers to reveal the crystals to the eastward direction. Chant:

> *"Good morning, East. I welcome you*
> *To bless with air energy these crystals two."*

Hold the crystals in your palms and soak in the eastern energy of air.

✦ Next, turn south and chant:

> *"Good morning, South. I welcome you*
> *To bless with fire energy these crystals two."*

Hold the crystals in your palms and soak in the southern energy of fire.

✦ Next, turn west and chant:

> *"Good morning, West. I welcome you*
> *To bless with water energy these crystals two."*

Hold the crystals in your palms and soak in the western energy of water.

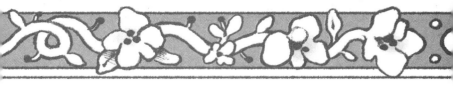

✦ Next, turn north and chant:

> *"Good morning, North. I welcome you*
> *To bless with earth energy these crystals two."*

Hold the crystals in your palms and soak in the northern energy of earth.

✦ Close your fingers back around the crystals and soak all that energy right to your core. Blow out the candle to seal the crystal energy to you. Carry your charged, blessed crystals with you for daylong energy.

POCKET FULL OF PROTECTION

PURPOSE OF SPELL: Magickally prevent illness by creating and carrying this protective charm.

SUGGESTED TIMING:
Full moon

ITEMS NEEDED:

- **2 small bowls**
- **Small** muslin bag or square of cloth
- **Twine** or string

MAGICKAL INGREDIENTS:

- 1 tablespoon dried parsley or 2 sprigs of fresh parsley
- 1 tablespoon dried rosemary or 2 sprigs of fresh rosemary
- 1 tourmaline crystal
- 1 smoky quartz crystal

SPELLWORK

✦ Lay out your ingredients on your altar. Place each of the herbs in their own small bowl. Place the tourmaline on top of the parsley and the smoky quartz on top of the rosemary. Seal their union by making a pentagram with your finger in the air above each pairing.

✦ Hold out both hands, palms down, one over each bowl, and incant:

> *"By darkness of parsley and by rosemary's light*
> *Seal these herbs, draw out their might*
> *The stones I bid to defend and protect*
> *Now into my bag, this magick collects."*

✦ Place all herbs and crystals in the bag or in the center of the strip of cloth. Using the string, tie the bag/cloth closed with three full knots while chanting:

> *"By knot of one, it is done.*
> *By knot of two, it will hold true.*
> *By knot of three, so mote it be."*

✦ Carry this magickal sachet with you, perhaps in your pocket or a purse, whenever you need protection from illness. Refresh ingredients and repeat as needed during each full moon.

THE BEND AND SNAP BACK

PURPOSE OF SPELL: This ritual is designed to beat fatigue and give you an energy boost on those days you need to keep going. Channel your inner Elle Woods, expert at perky manifestation, with this peppy ritual.

SUGGESTED TIMING:
Any time you need an energy boost, particularly midafternoon

ITEMS NEEDED:

- Essential oil diffuser
- Candle
- Lighter

MAGICKAL INGREDIENTS:

- Essential oil blend:
  3 drops peppermint oil,
  2 drops lemon oil,
  2 drops rosemary oil

SPELLWORK

✦ Add your essential oils to your diffuser.

✦ Light an unscented candle and center yourself. Notice the aroma of the essential oils. Focus on places you are holding stress in your body or where your body feels worn thin. Let the aroma seep into those places and start to gently energize them.

✦ Take five large, deep inhales and exhales.

✦ On each inhale, raise your arms high overhead. Extend them as far as your fingertips will reach, feeling your shoulders rise and your chest expand fully. Even get up on your tiptoes if it feels right.

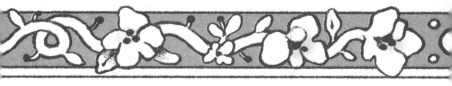

✦ As you exhale, bend forward at the waist, reaching your hands toward the floor. Do not worry about how far you can reach; this is not a yoga pose but a ritual movement—the simple yin and yang action of opening stretch to closing collapse is designed to align your energy for this spell.

✦ On your last inhale, come to a resting standing position and focus on your candle. Welcome the oils to fully refresh your aligned body. Feel your energy rise as the candle burns intently on. After a few minutes, blow out the candle, turn off the diffuser, and return to your busy day with more energy and drive.

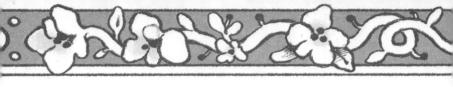

AN APPLE A DAY

PURPOSE OF SPELL: This spell is to help you maintain better nutrition to power your body for healing work.

SUGGESTED TIMING:
First thing in the morning or just before bedtime

ITEMS NEEDED:
- Athame
- 1 whole apple

MAGICKAL INGREDIENTS:
- ½ teaspoon cayenne pepper
- 1 green aventurine stone
- 1 citrine stone
- 3 drops cedar oil

SPELLWORK

✦ Place the apple on your altar. Place the aventurine crystal on one side of the apple and the citrine crystal on the other side of the apple.

✦ Stand with your feet firmly planted, hands over the apple, and incant:

*"Strength from within, strength from without
Make healthy choices, remove my self-doubt."*

✦ Cut the apple in half with your athame and say:

*"I sever this fruit with the will of my heart
To calm my cravings and gift myself a fresh start."*

✦ Anoint the apple with a few drops of cedar oil and say:

> *"As apple tree springs from the earth*
> *So shall my healthy appetite rebirth."*

✦ Sprinkle cayenne over the apple flesh and say:

> *"Quicken my healthy eating routine*
> *Avoiding sugars and replacing with greens."*

✦ Rub the two halves of the apple together deosil and say:

> *"By the energies born here I will it for me*
> *To make healthy choices, so mote it be."*

✦ Bury the apple halves outside, facedown, to seal the spell and increase your willpower over unhealthy temptations.

BEHIND THE MASK

PURPOSE OF SPELL: This spell will help you reveal your most authentic self through a facial skin refresh. Our most authentic self is our healthiest self. Yet we often wear masks of inauthenticity to conform to societal expectations. Use this facemask to refresh your visage and allow your true, beautiful self to shine bright.

SUGGESTED TIMING:
Waning moon, new moon

ITEMS NEEDED:

- Bowl
- Pestle and mortar
- Honey
- Water or cream

MAGICKAL INGREDIENTS:

- Ground turmeric
- 1 clear quartz stone
- 1 jasper stone

SPELLWORK

✦ Mix 1 teaspoon of turmeric powder with 1 tablespoon of honey.

✦ Slowly add enough heavy cream to smooth out the mixture. Stop when desired consistency is reached—usually when it's firm enough to easily scoop with your fingers but pliable enough to spread. Water is fine to substitute if you don't have cream.

✦ Hold the quartz in one hand and jasper in the other, and wave over the mixture in a back-and-forth motion.

✦ Incant:

> *"By red stone of jasper this red root of earth*
> *Shall uncover and activate my hidden self-worth.*
> *Honey shall sweeten the sting of those who reject my truth*
> *Cream returns my outlook to the hope of my youth."*

✦ Apply the mask to your face, and allow the rooted energy of turmeric and jasper to strip away anything attached to you that is not authentic. Allow it to set for 15 minutes. Promise yourself to be the person you are, even if that person bothers other people.

✦ Remove the mask with warm water, understanding this is how you heal. This is how you step into your power with the glow of self-confidence and leave the mess of masking behind. So mote it be.

KNOT TODAY, PAIN!

PURPOSE OF SPELL: This spell uses knot magick to draw the energy of pain out from the body and return it for healing to Mother Earth.

SUGGESTED TIMING:
As needed

ITEMS NEEDED:

- 6 to 8 inches of string, twine, or fabric strip
- Cauldron
- Long lighter

MAGICKAL INGREDIENTS:

- 1 tablespoon dried parsley
- ½ teaspoon garlic powder
- 1 black tourmaline crystal

SPELLWORK

✦ Loosely wrap your string around the tourmaline. The tourmaline will act as an agent to help draw out the pain from your body and into the string.

✦ Center your attention on the source of your pain. Place the tourmaline on the pain and chant:

> *"Pain be gone into this knot*
> *I draw you out of this very spot*
> *Heal me, mend me, set me free*
> *Be gone now pain, so mote it be."*

✦ Tie a knot in one end of the string. Repeat the placement and the chant.

✦ Tie a knot in the other end of the string. Repeat the placement and the chant.

✦ Remove the string from the tourmaline, and knot it directly in the middle.

✦ Add the parsley to your cauldron, and place the string on top of the parsley.

✦ Sprinkle the garlic powder on top of the parsley and string.

✦ Using the long lighter, set the cauldron contents on fire, burning them until they reduce to ash. As you burn, incant:

> *"As these knots burn, the pain is released
> Wellness is restored and suffering is ceased."*

✦ Bury the ashes outside in the earth or flush them down the toilet to rid yourself of these painful energies.

FERTILITY BOWL MAGICK

PURPOSE OF SPELL: This water bowl spell invokes the Mother Goddess magick of healing waters. The bowl in this spell represents the womb. The ingredients and method are meant to open the womb to the possibility of conception by removing any energetic blockages to that end.

SUGGESTED TIMING:
New moon

ITEMS NEEDED:
- Cauldron
- Boiling water

MAGICKAL INGREDIENTS:
- ½ cup sage leaf
- ¼ cup whole clove
- 2 tablespoons rosemary
- ¼ cup dried lavender buds
- Carnelian crystals
- Smoky quartz crystals
- Clear quartz crystals

SPELLWORK

✦ Add all herbs to the cauldron. Next, arrange your stones on top of the herbs in a circle. The carnelian will direct the herbs' power to the reproductive organs, and the quartzes will amplify this aid.

✦ Hold your hands over the bowl and incant:

> *"Sage for full body cleansing*
> *Clove for fertility increase*
> *Rosemary for Mother Goddess strength*
> *Lavender for inner warmth and peace."*

✦ Pour the boiling water over the herbs and stones until the bowl is almost full.

✦ Carefully place your face into the cooling steam and inhale the magick aroma into your lungs. Feel your lungs fill with healing light. Feel the crystals directing this healing light to the womb. Continue to breathe in the healing magick and breathe out anything blocking conception.

✦ As the water cools, know the magick is settling into your body to do its work. Discard the cooled water onto your plants for their magickal nourishment. Sleep with the magickally charged crystals nearby until the full moon to seal the spell.

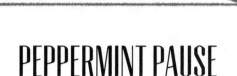

PEPPERMINT PAUSE

PURPOSE OF SPELL: This spell helps relieve tension headaches to get you back on track and on with your day.

SUGGESTED TIMING:
As needed

ITEMS NEEDED:
- Carrier oil, if desired

MAGICKAL INGREDIENTS:
- 1 clear quartz crystal
- 3 drops peppermint oil

SPELLWORK

✦ Begin this ritual by changing your location. Go outside if possible. Find a quiet stairwell in your office building if need be. Just move your body to a location different from where the headache started. Removing yourself from the tension vibe helps your body reset.

✦ Apply one drop of peppermint oil to each of your temples, mixing with carrier oil if desired.

✦ While massaging the peppermint into your temples, incant:

> *"Headache be gone, headache go free*
> *Do my bid and leave me be."*

✦ Next, apply a dab of oil to the nape of your neck. Repeat incantation.

THE HEALING POWER OF WITCHCRAFT

✦ Third, press the crystal to your forehead and repeat the incantation.

✦ Take three deep inhales and exhales to let the oil and crystals heal your pain into release.

✦ Repeat in an hour or as needed.

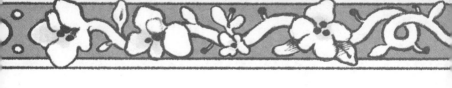

THE NAIL TRIM CURE

PURPOSE OF SPELL: This spell is meant to help your body overcome lingering illness and turn the tide of your energy toward robust health.

SUGGESTED TIMING:
Waning moon

ITEMS NEEDED:

- Cotton balls
- Nail trimmer
- Small glass jar or biodegradable bag

MAGICKAL INGREDIENTS:

- 1 tourmaline crystal
- 1 fluorite crystal
- Eucalyptus essential oil or tea tree oil (whichever scent you prefer, as needed)

SPELLWORK

✦ Close your eyes. Hold the tourmaline in one fist and fluorite in the other. Take at least 5 minutes to sit with the stones. These are absorbing stones, so focus on sending your negative energy and illness into them. Imagine all illness traveling from your body, down your arms, and into your fingernails and stones. Let it all collect into the stone and the very tips of your fingernails. When ready, release the stones to your altar to be cleansed and charged after the spell.

✦ Dab your preferred oil lightly on a cotton ball. Anoint each of your fingernails with the oil by using the cotton ball.

✦ Chant these lines, one for each finger:

"By power of one my illness is done
By power of two I have seen it through
By power of three I return to healthy
By power of four I feel poorly no more
By power of five I feel much more alive
By power of six my health I do fix
By power of seven my health is given
By power of eight no longer I wait
By power of nine health is mine
By power of ten so it is, amen."

✦ Trim your nails one by one, taking care to save the clippings.
Repeat the above incantation for each nail as you trim. Place
all the clippings in the jar or bag. Scatter them outside or bury
them if able, and let the illness release back into the earth for
healing.

HEALING MOON WATER ELIXIR

PURPOSE OF SPELL: Create a healing moon water elixir to add to your morning coffee or cooking for an infusion of health-drawing energy.

SUGGESTED TIMING:
Full moon

ITEMS NEEDED:
- Glass jar or bottle
- Fresh water

MAGICKAL INGREDIENTS:
- 1 green aventurine crystal
- 1 amethyst crystal
- 1 clear quartz crystal

SPELLWORK

✦ Fill your bottle with fresh water after sunset on the night of a full moon. Place the bottle on your altar along with three small crystals of green aventurine, amethyst, and clear quartz.

✦ Enchant your crystals with healing intention. Rub your hands together until they warm from friction, and hold your hands over the crystals, palms down. Imagine the heat flowing from your palms to the crystals is full of calm and healing.

✦ Add the green aventurine to the water and say:

"Stone of green, I call on thee
Keep me strong and illness free."

✦ Add the amethyst to the water and say:

> *"Stone of purple, I call on thee*
> *Soothe my mind and heal my body."*

✦ Add the clear quartz to the water and say:

> *"Stone of universal energy,*
> *Amplify my intent, so mote it be."*

✦ Close the bottle securely. Swirl the ingredients in the closed bottle deosil three times to bind all energies together.

✦ Place the water/crystal mixture out under the moonlight to magickally charge. Be sure to bring in the newly created Moon Water elixir before dawn. Store in a shaded, cool cupboard and avoid placing in direct sunlight. Use a drop or two daily in your beverage of choice or cooking to infuse your body with this magickal healing elixir.

SEXY SPARK SPELL

PURPOSE OF SPELL: Perform this crystal and candle magick spell prior to lovemaking with self or partner to heal you from a sexual rut, increase libido, and inspire passion.

SUGGESTED TIMING:
Waxing moon, full moon

ITEMS NEEDED:

- Essential oil diffuser
- Candle
- Small heat-safe bowl filled with salt
- Lighter

MAGICKAL INGREDIENTS:

- 1 teaspoon cayenne
- 1 teaspoon cinnamon
- 1 jasper crystal
- 1 carnelian crystal
- 1 rose quartz crystal
- 1 citrine crystal
- Essential oil blend:
  2 drops basil,
  2 drops ylang-ylang,
  2 drops rosemary,
  2 drops cedarwood

SPELLWORK

✦ Add your oil blend to your diffuser and turn on.

✦ Put on some music and/or clothing that makes you feel sexy if you desire. You might even want to enjoy a glass of wine. This is a spell of joyfully raised sex energy, so use any method that makes you open to lust and passion.

✦ Set your altar with your ingredients. Place jasper toward the north, place carnelian toward the south, place rose quartz

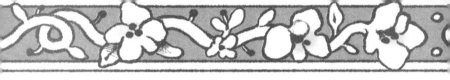

toward the east, and place citrine toward the west. These are all sex and love crystals, and they will create a vortex of passion on your altar. Place your bowl of salt in the center of the four crystal crossroads. Heap the cayenne and cinnamon on top of the salt. Nestle the candle securely in the middle of the mixture.

✦ Light the candle and enchant your senses by the light of the dancing flame. Chant:

> *"My eyes receive beauty in shapely body*
> *My nose smells lust on my lover's neck*
> *My ears hear soft breathing quickening*
> *My fingers graze to pleasure zones*
> *My lips taste passion with every kiss."*

✦ Continue to move your body to the music, taking in the scent of the room. When you feel the energy turn to tension, blow out the candle and embrace the pleasures of release ahead.

CUNNING THE COMMON COLD

PURPOSE OF SPELL: This spell is a traditional, calming hearth witch steam and potion for those days you are down and out with the common cold.

SUGGESTED TIMING:
As needed

ITEMS NEEDED:

- Medium kitchen pot filled with water
- Teacup
- Athame
- Towel

MAGICKAL INGREDIENTS:

- 1 smoky quartz crystal
- Get-well potion:
  ½ teaspoon minced garlic,
  pinch of cayenne,
  1 teaspoon fresh ginger,
  2 tablespoons lemon juice,
  ½ teaspoon cinnamon,
  1 teaspoon honey if desired
- Essential oil blend:
  4 drops eucalyptus,
  3 drops peppermint oil,
  2 drops rosemary oil

SPELLWORK

✦ Set the pot of water to boil on your stove.

✦ Charge your towel with calming vibes by wrapping it around the smoky quartz. Set the towel out of the way, but in arm's reach.

✦ Prepare your potion. Whisk together the garlic, lemon juice, and ginger in a small bowl. Mix in the cayenne and cinnamon.

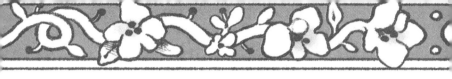

When well mixed, transfer the potion to a teacup. Press the point of your ceremonial knife or athame into the center of the potion.

✦ Hold the athame firm and chant:

"With this knife, I cut in two
The power of this cold and flu
Let this potion disperse my ill
So it is, this is my will."

✦ When the water has boiled, remove it from the hot burner and fill your teacup with boiling water. Place the rest of the potted water on a cool burner, and add the essential oil blend.

✦ Carefully place your face in the steam of the pot of boiling water, making sure it is not too hot before proceeding. Cover your head with the towel to help direct the steam to your face. The water will continue to steam for a bit, and you will inhale this medicinal steam. On the inhale, concentrate on the healing energies entering your throat, lungs, and chest. On the exhale, release your illness out of your body to be purified in the steam. Repeat until the steam has cooled. Dry your face with the towel. Dump the cooled water, and your illness, down the drain to discard.

✦ Finally, drink your cooled healing potion. Add a bit of honey on the rim of your teacup before drinking, if desired. Hold your smoky quartz for healing company as you do. Cleanse your palate with a little dark chocolate if needed. Climb into bed with a good book and get some rest.

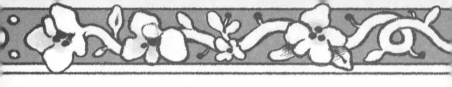

SLEEPYTIME CANDLE MAGICK

PURPOSE OF SPELL: This spell will help you rest better throughout the night by harnessing the calming power of lavender, sage, amethyst, and essential oils through the energy work of candle magick.

SUGGESTED TIMING:
Before bedtime

ITEMS NEEDED:

- 1 candle
- Lighter
- 1 plate
- Cauldron filled with 2 inches of salt
- 1 small muslin bag or cloth square

MAGICKAL INGREDIENTS:

- ¼ cup dried lavender
- 1 teaspoon ground sage
- 1 amethyst crystal
- 1 smoky quartz crystal
- Lavender, ylang-ylang, jasmine, or vanilla essential oil (choose based on the scent you most prefer for calming vibes)

SPELLWORK

✦ Begin by mixing the lavender and sage together and spread the mixture on a plate. Draw a pentagram with your finger in the mixture to charge it.

✦ Anoint the candle with your chosen oil.

✦ Dress the oiled candle in the mixture, coating the candle in the herbs. Nestle the newly dressed candle in the middle of the salt-filled cauldron. Scrape the remaining herbs into the muslin bag.

✦ Place the bag and the two crystals in front of the candle. The energy of the burning candle will charge them to their full sleep-inducing potential.

✦ When ready, light the candle and incant:

> *"The candle is lit, the day is done,*
> *I count backwards from ten to one."*

✦ Sit comfortably in front of the candle. Focus on the dancing flame, or close your eyes and bask in the candlelight, whichever feels more relaxing to you.

✦ Take a large inhale; allow your chest to swell with air. Hold for 3 seconds. In these 3 seconds, focus on nothing. Let your mind clear completely. Next, exhale completely, speaking the number "ten" at the end of your exhale. Repeat this process. Begin with your next big inhale, then hold for 3 seconds, exhale, and say "nine." Continue down through "one."

✦ The goal is to slow your body. Think of it as a release from the day. Give yourself the gift of time spent doing nothing but breathing. Allow for the slowed flow to penetrate and heal your restlessness.

✦ When ready, blow out the candle and incant:

> *"The spell is done, so mote it be,*
> *Restful sleep shall come to me."*

✦ Bring your sachet of herbs and two crystals to your nightstand or place them under your pillow to keep the restful energy near you all night long.

TRIPLE GODDESS POWER

PURPOSE OF SPELL: This spell recharges and renews your **body.** The Goddess archetype is referred to as the Triple Goddess when honoring the three stages of the feminine life cycle: maiden, mother, and crone. Regardless of specific religious belief, there remains great magickal energy in harnessing the natural power cycle of youth, fertility, and old age. Invoke the three powerful facets of the Triple Goddess archetype to recharge and renew your body.

SUGGESTED TIMING:
New moon, waxing moon

ITEMS NEEDED:

* 3 candles
* Lighter

MAGICKAL INGREDIENTS:

* ¼ teaspoon powdered ginger

SPELLWORK

✦ Begin by sprinkling the powdered ginger lightly over the candles to invoke invigorating healing energy.

✦ Incant:

> *"As I light these candles three*
> *I call the powers of Goddess to me*
> *Recharge and renew my body in full*
> *Give me strength, make me whole."*

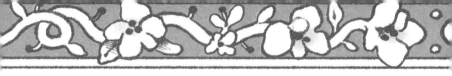

✦ Light the first candle and say:

>*"This first flame for the Maiden,*
>*Her boundless youth rejuvenates my body."*

✦ Light the second candle and say:

>*"This second flame for the Mother*
>*Her guiding touch gifts me loving renewal."*

✦ Light the third candle and say:

>*"This third flame for the Crone*
>*Her steadfast wisdom recharges my bones.*
>*Goddess grant these divine gifts to me.*
>*I will use them in love and in honor of thee.*
>*It is done, so mote it be."*

✦ Sit with your candles, soaking in the love of the Goddess. When ready, blow them out and engage your day, knowing the power of the Goddess has renewed your body.

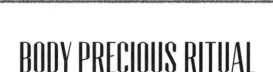

BODY PRECIOUS RITUAL

PURPOSE OF SPELL: This spell is for body positivity and connects you with your physical body using gratitude and love. By flooding your body parts with gratitude, you encourage your body to flourish and heal, turning self-depreciation into self-appreciation.

SUGGESTED TIMING:
Whenever you are feeling low on self-esteem or disconnected from self-love

ITEMS NEEDED:
• Essential oil diffuser

MAGICKAL INGREDIENTS:
• 1 rose quartz crystal
• 1 green aventurine crystal
• Essential oil blend:
  3 drops rosemary oil,
  3 drops orange oil,
  2 drops bergamot

SPELLWORK

✦ Sit in a quiet, comfortable location with your oil blend working in the diffuser. Hold the rose quartz stone in one hand and the green aventurine stone in the other. Make a fist around the stones.

✦ Take slow, relaxing breaths while concentrating on the loving power of rose quartz and the heart-healing powers of green aventurine. Imagine the stones sending pulsating energy up your arms and into your core. Feel the health and love energies intertwine and figure-eight throughout your body.

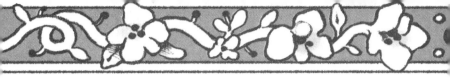

✦ When ready, chant:

"I am more resilient than I realize,
I am stronger than I feel,
I am smarter than I think,
I am more beautiful than I imagine,
I am healing."

✦ Repeat three times. Sleep with the stones under your pillow that night to fully soak in the healing love.

4

HEAL YOUR MIND

The mind is one of the most powerful components of magickal healing. By learning to soothe our irritated egos with knowledge, fresh perspective, and release, we replace negative emotions and energy with higher, more helpful modes of operating. Emotions like doubt, jealousy, fear, hate, anger, and apathy disperse with the application of the healing power of intentional love. The spells that follow are crafted to help you find peace of mind so you may heal and thus produce a higher, more magickal energy, flowing toward the greater good.

CRYSTAL CAIRN MAGICK

PURPOSE OF SPELL: This ritual is designed to help you ground and find balance and prepare your mind for necessary healing. Cairns are balanced, man-made piles of rocks used by our ancient ancestors as guides for travelers and as denotation of magickal spaces. Apply this ancient practice of building a cairn by using your crystals to invoke a grounded balance in your magickal space.

SUGGESTED TIMING:
As needed

ITEMS NEEDED:
• Flat, calm surface

MAGICKAL INGREDIENTS:
• 4 to 5 crystals of your choosing

SPELLWORK

✦ Select crystals from your collection that lend themselves to balanced stacking. Usually the flatter the crystal the better. If you do not have many stackable crystals, it is equally as magickal to forage in your local natural environments for flat rocks that can serve the same balancing purpose. Usually beaches and streams produce excellent flat rocks due to the wear of water on their shapes. Perhaps a mix of crystal and local rocks will be the most effective for you!

CONTINUED >>>

✦ Arrange the stones in a line on your altar from largest to smallest, left to right. Now, carefully and patiently place the smaller crystals or stones on top of the larger ones. Notice how the solid foundation allows for upward mobility. Feel the balance of smaller crystals depending on larger ones for support. Consider how foundations and support work in your own life. Where do you need more of each?

✦ As you contemplate, bless your cairn with the following incantation:

> *"Stones of balance and harmony*
> *Help my mind with stability*
> *Building steady toward the sky*
> *With sturdy foundations as my guide."*

✦ When ready, leave your cairn to work its grounding magick and serve as a reminder to return to your authentic foundation when you are feeling out of sorts.

WORRIED WEAVER'S CHARM

PURPOSE OF SPELL: This spell uses the powers of healing spices and weaving magick to draw calming vibes to the anxious mind.

SUGGESTED TIMING:
Waxing moon, full moon

ITEMS NEEDED:

- 3 ribbons or strips of cloth cut into 12-by-2-inch pieces. An old T-shirt will work well for this.
- Large heat-safe bowl
- Boiling water

MAGICKAL INGREDIENTS:

- 1 teaspoon ground sage
- 1 teaspoon ground clove
- 1 teaspoon ground anise
  (use a tablespoon of each if using fresh sage leaf, whole cloves, or star anise)

SPELLWORK

✦ Set out the three strips of ribbon or cloth next to your heat-safe bowl on your altar.

✦ Add the sage, clove, and anise to the bowl. When ready, pour the boiling water into the bowl over the herbs to activate their powers. While the water is steaming, add each strip of cloth to the bowl one by one.

CONTINUED >>>

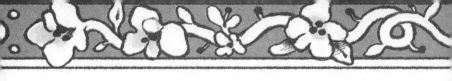

✦ Incant:

> "This first ribbon is for protection,
> Keep me safe and free of harm.
>
> This second ribbon is for serenity,
> Soothe my fears and keep me calm.
>
> This third ribbon is for mental strength,
> Aid me with self-confidence and
> Dispel my anxious qualms."

✦ **Allow** the ribbons to soak in the magick of the spices until **the water** cools. Enjoy the calming scent of the herbs as they **give off** their healing energy.

✦ Once the three ribbons are cooled, braid or twist them **together** to bind the spell.

✦ Set the ribbons to dry on your altar overnight.

✦ Wear or carry the braided charm to combat anxiety.

THE HEALING POWER OF WITCHCRAFT

THE WITCH'S JAR

PURPOSE OF SPELL: This spell uses the banishing magick of the traditional witch's jar to contain and assuage anger. Anger causes disservice to healing, even if our anger is justified. Anger can make us say or do things we don't really mean or that do not align with our healing mission. Assuaging anger is even healing in and of itself, considering the peace it brings. Use this jar spell to calm anger so you may move forward with clarity to address the situation.

SUGGESTED TIMING:
As needed

ITEMS NEEDED:

- Medium-sized jar with lid
- A handful of sharp objects like thumbtacks, pins, or nails
- Candle and lighter for hot liquid wax

MAGICKAL INGREDIENTS:

- 2 tablespoons oregano
- 2 tablespoons chamomile
- 1 tourmaline crystal
- 1 jasper crystal

SPELLWORK

✦ Place the individual sharp objects in the jar one by one. As you drop each one, think about the reasons you are angry. Really put your energy into the words or actions that hurt you. Let it all out with the careful handling of sharp, scary objects. Think about how carefully handling anger is a protective move for your health.

CONTINUED >>>

✦ Next, add the oregano to the jar for peace and release, and the chamomile for a calming effect.

✦ Third, place the stones on top of the herbs. The tourmaline will absorb the anger, and the jasper will ground and even your emotions.

✦ Use the lighter to melt off wax from the candle, then close the lid and seal the jar with the wax. Bury this witch's jar of banished anger outside to let earth magick absorb and banish the anger so you may proceed with clarity and heal from the detrimental effects of anger. Dig up the jar in 3 days and retrieve the crystals to charge them. Discard the remaining contents with your anger in an outside bin.

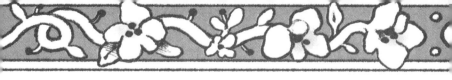

MISTY LIFTING SPRAY

PURPOSE OF SPELL: Depression can be all-consuming and crippling. Even seemingly small tasks like showering can seem insurmountable. To help pull yourself out of the dark and toward the light, use this ritual mist to freshen your blankets, sheets, clothes, body, or hair without much effort. Make this when you are feeling well to give yourself a boost on days when you cannot muster much energy to do anything.

SUGGESTED TIMING:
Craft under the full moon, use as needed

ITEMS NEEDED:

- Empty, clean, fine mist spray bottle
- 1 ounce distilled water
- 1 ounce hydrosol or vodka

MAGICKAL INGREDIENTS:

- Smoky quartz crystals
- Rose quartz crystals
- Essential oil blend:
  8 drops ylang-ylang oil,
  8 drops bergamot oil,
  8 drops orange oil

SPELLWORK

✦ Combine the water and alcohol in the spray bottle. Swirl gently to mix the ingredients.

✦ Add the oils to the bottle. Again, swirl and roll the bottle to mix thoroughly.

CONTINUED >>>

✦ Set the bottle out under the full moon, surrounded by the quartz crystals. Let the full moon energy charge the crystals and the mixture all together, magickally binding their depression-relieving properties.

✦ Store the bottle in a cool, shaded location for up to a month of use. Spray as needed on your clothes, bedsheets, couch, or hair to lift your mood and help you feel refreshed.

STRESS BALL CHARM

PURPOSE OF SPELL: Reduce stress by crafting this stress ball charm and displaying it in your home or on your altar.

SUGGESTED TIMING:
Craft under a waning moon

ITEMS NEEDED:

- Essential oil diffuser
- 1 large orange
- Toothpick
- Plate
- Crafting wire (Yule ornament hook or even a paperclip should work)
- String or ribbon
- Small jar

MAGICKAL INGREDIENTS:

- Design: ½ cup whole cloves
- Potion:
  1 teaspoon cinnamon,
  1 teaspoon ground clove,
  1 teaspoon nutmeg,
  1 piece of smoky quartz
- Essential oil blend:
  2 drops lavender,
  2 drops bergamot,
  1 drop orange,
  2 drops ylang-ylang

SPELLWORK

✦ Turn on your essential oil diffuser with the blend in it.

✦ Using the pointy end, push the whole cloves into the orange to create aromatic, stress-relieving designs or sigils. You may want to pre-puncture the holes with your toothpick to create the design and then add the cloves to the holes after the design

CONTINUED >>>

is complete. Create whatever design feels right to you. Some options are hearts, stars, diamonds, lines, arrows, or a letter.

✦ Meanwhile, ready your potion by mixing the spices and spreading the mixture out on a plate.

✦ When the orange and clove design is done, roll the orange over the potion mixture on the plate. Notice the juices released by the skin punctures will help the spices really stick to the orange. Let the orange sit for a few moments in the potion.

✦ Remove the orange and pierce the skin with the wire, running the wire under a sturdy patch of skin and out again. Attach the string to the wire. Hang the charm from a doorknob or curtain rod where it will emanate antistress vibes. Discard when the orange begins to turn white.

✦ Bonus! Save the excess potion in a jar. Add a smoky quartz crystal to activate the potion. You can keep the jar on your altar, in your glove compartment, by your bed, in a drawer at work— wherever you need a little more stress relief in your life.

MOON HEALING FOR THE BROKEN HEART

PURPOSE OF SPELL: Broken hearts hurt like hell. There is no doubt about that. With great pain, the fix is never instantaneous, but consistent healing work truly helps. This spell is an effective way to use the moon cycle to release your past lover out of your life and move on in confidence and in love.

SUGGESTED TIMING:
Identify the dates of the next new moon, waxing moon, full moon, and waning moon. You are going to perform this spell on each of those nights with a progressive end of healing and release.

ITEMS NEEDED:
- Cauldron
- Scissors
- Small jar

ITEMS CONT.
- Three 6-inch pieces of string
- Long lighter
- A photograph of you and your ex

MAGICKAL INGREDIENTS:
- 1 sodalite crystal
- 1 jasper crystal
- 1 fluorite crystal
- 1 rose quartz crystal

SPELLWORK

✦ On the night of the new moon, the spell's focus will be addressing the breakup so you may start anew.

CONTINUED >>>

✦ Begin by ripping the photograph in half with you on one side and your ex on the other. Place the halves on your altar and connect the two pieces with a string. Hold the sodalite, stone of verbal expression and peace, in one hand. Place your index finger on the string. Imagine your ex standing in front of you. Tell them everything you need to. Maybe you yell at them, maybe you sob, maybe you tell them you love them. Speak whatever truth is real for you as you feel it toward them. When done, cut the string and save it in the jar along with the photograph and the sodalite. Let the sodalite work its calming, truth-filled magick on the severed string and photo.

✦ Next up is the night of the waxing moon. Repeat the same spread on your altar with the torn photograph from the jar with a new string between the two halves. Hold the jasper, the stone of grounding and rootedness, in your hand. Place your finger on the string and think about all the things you have done for yourself in the past week and can continue to do. Return to your own roots. Consider making art, cooking, or writing. Find a place to start again in the foundations of your own strengths and talents. When done, cut the string and save it in the jar along with the other strings, the photograph, and the jasper. Let the jasper root you in a new beginning.

✦ Next comes the night of the full moon. Repeat the same spread on your altar with the torn picture from the jar with a new string between the two halves. Hold fluorite, the stone of purging and cleansing, in your hand. Place your finger on the string and tell your ex-lover everything you reject about them.

Focus on the things that hurt you or were not healthy for you. Get it all out into the string and fluorite for a full release of those negative energies. You deserve nothing but positive vibes. When done, cut the string and save it in the jar along with the other strings, the photograph, and the fluorite. Let the fluorite cleanse the bad energy of the relationship from your past so you may move forward free of low vibes.

✦ Finally comes the night of the waning moon. Look how far you have come, witch! Time to take all your strings and the half photo of your ex. Burn them together in your cauldron, reducing them to ash. A long lighter works well for this, as you can hold the flame directly on the items. As you burn, hold the rose quartz in your hand. Feel the past release. Transfer this relief to the rose quartz in the form of self-love. Release your lover for the final time and step forward in self-confident love and optimism for the future. Carry the rose quartz on you until the new moon when the spell will be complete.

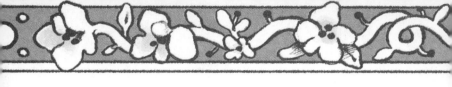

RINGS A BELL

PURPOSE OF SPELL: This charm is designed to help heal a failing memory, improve your memory, and help retain information.

SUGGESTED TIMING:
Waxing moon, full moon

ITEMS NEEDED:

- Bell
- Small bowl of warm water
- Candle
- Small muslin bag

MAGICKAL INGREDIENTS:

- 1 teaspoon ground cinnamon
- 1 tablespoon whole clove
- 1 amethyst crystal
- 1 clear quartz crystal

SPELLWORK

✦ Light the candle next to the bowl of warm water. Did you know water has memory? Since water is recycled through the natural cycles of evaporation and condensation, it is a powerful agent of steadfastness. Use this knowledge as you swirl your finger deosil in the water three times to charge it by the light of the candle.

✦ Ring your bell three times.

✦ Add the cinnamon, clove, and crystals to the water.

✦ Ring your bell again three times.

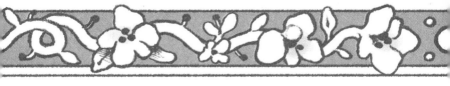

✦ Let the candle burn for at least an hour as the ingredients fully charge.

✦ When the energy feels maxed, ring the bell three more times.

✦ Drain the water from the bowl and keep the crystals and spices. Place them in the muslin bag and leave to dry beneath the light of the full moon. Touch and smell the charm bag whenever you need a boost in your memory skills. Place it on your desk as you work or study. Let the magick heal your scattered brain and help you retain information.

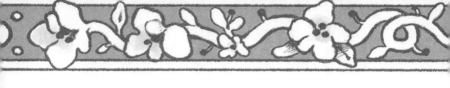

HAPPINESS BY THE JARFUL

PURPOSE OF SPELL: This jar spell is a powerful way to create happy and optimistic energy when you are feeling down. This is healing magick you can return to and use as needed.

SUGGESTED TIMING:
Full moon

ITEMS NEEDED:

- Empty mason or pickle jar filled with 2 inches of salt
- Small candle
- Lighter

MAGICKAL INGREDIENTS:

- 3 tablespoons chamomile
- 5 sprigs of fresh mint
- 1 citrine crystal
- 1 carnelian crystal
- 3 drops orange oil

SPELLWORK

✦ Add the chamomile on top of the salt, and arrange the sprigs of mint around the edge of the jar. Place the citrine and carnelian in the jar as well.

✦ Anoint the candle with the orange oil while incanting:

> *"Scent of happy, bring joyous cheer,*
> *Burn away sadness, burn away fear."*

✦ Nestle the candle in the center of the salt.

✦ When ready, light the candle and incant:

"Jar of optimism, bountiful and fierce
By this light all gloom doth pierced.
I stand witness to the growing cheer
And harness its essence for use all year."

✦ Allow the candle to burn below the rim of the jar if it hasn't already. Blow out the candle, and quickly close the lid to capture some of the candle smoke in the jar.

✦ This jar will emanate happy vibes, so pick a visible place for it. Perhaps it fits well near the kitchen sink while you wash dishes or on your dresser to set the vibe as you get dressed in the morning.

✦ If you feel the jar go a bit stale, all you need to do is relight the candle for a few minutes under moonlight to charge. You may also replace the mint for a quick refresh and infusion of luck if you need it. Typically, the jar's powers last as long as the candle does, at which point you can make a new one on the next full moon if desired.

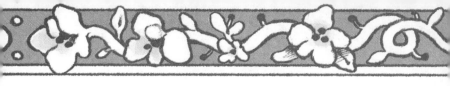

THE STRONGEST OF THEM ALL

PURPOSE OF SPELL: This spell harnesses your inner power to reveal and boost your healing strength by enchanting your mirror.

SUGGESTED TIMING:
Waxing moon, full moon

ITEMS NEEDED:

- Small bowl
- Jojoba oil
- Mirror
- Two 12-inch pieces of string or twine

MAGICKAL INGREDIENTS:

- 3 sprigs of rosemary
- 3 sprigs of thyme
- 7 drops tea tree oil or cedar oil (whichever scent you prefer for healing strength)

SPELLWORK

✦ Disperse 7 drops of your chosen oil in 1 tablespoon of carrier oil like jojoba oil. Place the oil mixture in a small bowl on your altar.

✦ Soak the two pieces of string in the oil mixture for at least an hour. Let the fortifying and strengthening properties of the oil really penetrate the string.

✦ When ready, take out the string and slide off excess oil by running it through your thumb and forefinger. Feel free to anoint your temples and nape of your neck with the excess oil if you desire a boost in grounding strength.

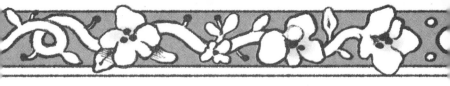

✦ Next, make two bundles of herbs. Tie the three sprigs of rosemary together with one of the strings to amplify your healing power. Tie the three sprigs of thyme together to bind strength to you.

✦ Now it is time to enchant your mirror. Take a sprig bundle in each hand.

✦ Wave the bundles in front of your mirror and all around it, incanting:

"Mirror mirror, reflection of mine
Enchanted with rosemary and with thyme
The witch in the mirror is me
A powerful healer, so mote it be."

✦ Hang your bundles from the corners of your mirror or place them at the base. As they dry, they will seal your mirror as an enchanted, magickally boosted projection of your inner power and healing strength, which you may access every time you look in the mirror.

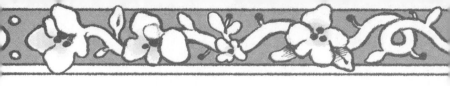

SOUL SPIRAL MAGICK

PURPOSE OF SPELL: This spell will help free and heal you from negative, toxic patterns that are holding you back from fully healing.

SUGGESTED TIMING:
Full moon, waning moon, new moon

ITEMS NEEDED:

- Candle
- Cauldron
- Pen and paper
- Long lighter

ITEMS CONT.

- Small bowl filled with an inch or two of salt
- Athame

MAGICKAL INGREDIENTS:

- ½ cup whole peppercorn or whole clove
- 1 tablespoon turmeric
- 1 fluorite crystal

SPELLWORK

✦ Begin by writing down the toxic patterns or people who are holding you back from fully healing.

✦ Light your candle. Incant:

> *"Burn and release, set me free*
> *Show me the most authentic me*
> *Remove fear and negativity*
> *Out toxic patterns, let me be!"*

✦ Burn the piece of paper in the candle flame, dropping it in your cauldron as the flame encroaches on your fingers. Finish

burning the paper if necessary with a long lighter. Set aside the cauldron with the ashes.

✦ Next, create the banishing potion. Take your bowl of salt and spread a layer of peppercorn or clove on top. Evenly sprinkle the turmeric over the mixture. Finally, top the mixture with a layer of the ash from your cauldron.

✦ Insert the point of your athame into the potion at the top left corner of the bowl. Slowly move your knife in a fluid spiral fashion, widdershins, or counterclockwise. Spiral increasingly closer to the center.

✦ Stop when you reach the center and incant:

"Spiral down, spiral out
Suck out these habits and self-doubt.
Spiral away, spiral stay
Move me, break me, refresh my way."

✦ Remove the athame. Seal your newly created spiral by placing the fluorite crystal in the center. Leave the magickal spiral on your altar to soak in negative toxic energy and remove it from your life. Discard by scattering the potion outside after 7 days and nights to complete the spell.

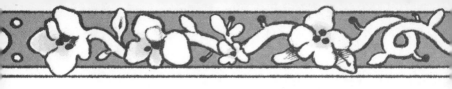

MISSION IMPOSTER HEALING

PURPOSE OF SPELL: The purpose of this spell is a ritual burn to alleviate the effects of imposter syndrome that hold you back from stepping into your truth and power.

Imposter syndrome is the internalized rejection of yourself as you are. It is the feeling of inadequacy, despite mounds of evidence to the contrary. Imposter syndrome is rampant in the witch community and for good reason. How many years of history have been spent beating down any reclamation of our power? How often have we been told magick isn't real, or if it is real, then it is surely evil? It is a constant battle for so many to hold our heads high and keep on witching. Here is how we can heal from that.

SUGGESTED TIMING:
Waxing moon, full moon

ITEMS NEEDED:

- Cauldron
- Small candle
- Salt

MAGICKAL INGREDIENTS:

- 1 tablespoon thyme
- 1 tablespoon oregano
- 3 citrine crystals
- 3 clear quartz crystals

SPELLWORK

✦ Fill your cauldron with a few inches of salt. Cover the salt with the thyme for strength and the oregano to release. The combination of inner strength and release of outer opinions will help heal you from the haunting doubts of imposter syndrome. Nestle the candle in the center of the cauldron.

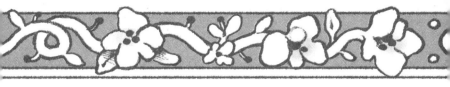

✦ Charge the mixture by surrounding the cauldron with citrine to bolster your sense of self and with clear quartz to amplify the energy.

✦ Light the candle and incant:

"I am a witch.
I reject doubt and I accept my truth.
I dispel negativity and I honor my own willpower.
I lean into my inner knowing and my magick.
See me heal.
See me fly.
I am a witch."

✦ Let the candle burn all the way down to the salt. Be careful not to leave it unattended while it burns. Perhaps you take this time to read some witchy books and work on your witchy knowledge base. Perhaps you meditate or do yoga. Use the time to self-improve in defiance of those who would see you fail. Once the candle is completely burned, know this energy transfer has healed your sense of self. You ARE a witch.

THE ZONE-IN POTION

PURPOSE OF SPELL: Create a magickal potion to heal a scattered brain and aid with focus and concentration when you need it.

SUGGESTED TIMING:
Create under a waxing or full moon; use as needed

ITEMS NEEDED:

- 3 tablespoons olive oil or grapeseed oil
- Small saucepan
- Cheese cloth
- Small mason jar

MAGICKAL INGREDIENTS:

- 3 cinnamon sticks
- 2 tablespoons dried lavender bud
- Essential oil blend:
  8 drops orange oil,
  4 drops peppermint oil,
  2 drops ylang-ylang oil

SPELLWORK

✦ Heat oil in the saucepan over medium heat until shimmery and viscous.

✦ Stir in the cinnamon sticks and lavender bud, simmer on low for 3 to 5 minutes.

✦ Stir occasionally.

✦ Remove from heat and let sit for another 3 to 5 minutes.

✦ Strain the cooling mixture through the cheesecloth and into the jar.

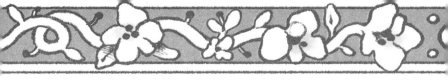

✦ Discard the cinnamon and buds outside as an offering to Mother Earth.

✦ Add the essential oils to the jar.

✦ Shake the potion well, repeating:

> *"Zone me in, zone the world out*
> *Keep my attention, release me from distraction*
> *I shake above, I shake below*
> *Mix well my potion, let focus grow."*

✦ Place the potion out under the waxing or full moon to charge. Dab some on your wrists, temples, or nape of your neck whenever you need to heal a lack of focus.

THE OREGANO ADJUSTMENT

PURPOSE OF SPELL: This spell will help you release unrealistic or toxic expectations of others that weigh down your sense of clarity and set you up for unnecessary disappointment. Heal your outlook with this release spell.

SUGGESTED TIMING:
Waning moon, new moon

ITEMS NEEDED:

- Cauldron
- Lighter

MAGICKAL INGREDIENTS:

- 1 sprig of dried oregano

SPELLWORK

✦ Hold the oregano sprig by one end just above your cauldron.

✦ Bless the oregano by incanting:

"Herb of grounding, herb of peace
Help me temper and release
What is will be
What was is done
Release the hold these thoughts have spun
I burn you now, so flame in haste
Baleful expectations are now erased."

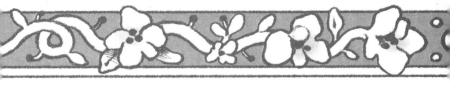

✦ Light the end of the oregano sprig. As the sprig burns, focus on readjusting your attitude to welcome understanding. Notice how just being with the homey aromatic scent calms and opens the soul. As the leaves shrivel in the fire, let anything holding you back from embracing healthy expectations release and burn away. Release the sprig into the cauldron once it nears your fingers. Gently inhale the remaining smoke to cleanse and finish the spell. As the smoke clears, so the spell is in effect.

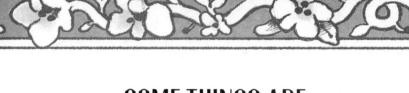

SOME THINGS ARE WORTH MELTING FOR

PURPOSE OF SPELL: This spell is to foster patience. The healing process is often long and winding, albeit rewarding. Some days are harder than others to latch on to the patience needed with yourself. Use this spell as a potent reminder that slow and steady wins the race.

SUGGESTED TIMING:
New moon, waxing moon

ITEMS NEEDED:

- Freezer-safe bowl or ice tray (silicone container is recommended, as it is easiest to work with)
- Candle
- Light

ITEMS CONT.

- Water
- Larger bowl

MAGICKAL INGREDIENTS:

- 1 tablespoon dried lavender
- 1 tablespoon dried rosemary
- 1 tablespoon dried thyme

SPELLWORK

✦ Secure your candle to the bottom of the bowl/ice tray. To do this, light a candle briefly and let the wax melt a bit. Drip the melting wax into the center of the bowl or ice tray and press your candle in it. Hold the candle in place, allowing the wax to cool and harden and secure your candle in place.

✦ Next, pour water into the bowl. As you do, imagine pouring your frustrations and worries out of your body and into the bowl.

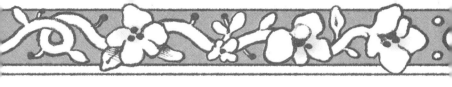

✦ Add your healing herbs to the water. As you add the lavender, invite calmness to heal your frustrations. As you add rosemary, invite love to soothe your worries. As you add thyme, invite strength and fortitude to be your forward guide.

✦ Carefully place the bowl or ice tray into the freezer. Make sure it is level so it will freeze evenly. Let freeze overnight as the herbs work their magick on your frustrations.

✦ In the morning, remove the ice potion from its container. Place the ice potion on your altar in a larger bowl to catch the water as it melts.

✦ Light your candle and chant three times:

> *"As this ice melts to liquid form*
> *I call my patience to be reborn.*
> *Let my frustrations diffuse and wane,*
> *Fleeting like the falling rain."*

✦ Once the ice is melted, pour the melted potion outside into the earth. Draw a pentagram on the wet spot in the earth with your finger. This will seal the spell with patient earth magick to help heal your impatience.

EYE OF THE BEHOLDER

PURPOSE OF SPELL: This ritual releases us from petty jealousies and gossip that sap our positive energy and leave us unable to address our own healing work.

SUGGESTED TIMING:
New moon

ITEMS NEEDED:
- Medium-sized bowl lined with 1 inch of salt

MAGICKAL INGREDIENTS:
- 1 cup whole cloves
- 1 tablespoon black pepper
- ½ cup dried lavender

SPELLWORK

✦ For this ritual, you are going to use your healing herbs and spices to create a charm to release you from a petty mindset and create an eye of compassion with which to see the world.

✦ Begin by crafting the outline of the eye in the bowl of salt. Make an oblong oval shape out of whole cloves. As you lay each tiny clove end to end, think about all the times you focused on insignificant slights or offenses instead of compassion or release. Think about those you are jealous of and why you feel that way. Clove absorbs our negative energies, so really get it all out.

✦ Chant as you craft:

"Clove upon clove, end to end, put my pettiness to mend."

✦ Next, add the pupil in the center of the eye by dumping the black pepper in a heap in the middle. Black pepper is a powerful release agent, so really let it accumulate in the center to help force out any lingering jealousies.

✦ Hold your hands over the pepper pupil and incant:

> *"Pepper quicken, set me free, no more petty jealousy."*

✦ Finally, design the iris of the eye with your lavender buds. Gently surround the pepper pupil with the calming, healing properties of lavender. Lavender is also a psychic opener, so it will help you use your intuition instead of your ego to judge situations.

✦ Incant:

> *"Lavender soothe my restless heart,*
> *Renew my sight with a fresh start."*

✦ Set your eye of compassionate clarity outside under the new moon to activate its power and fully allow your release.

HEAL YOUR SPIRIT

T he witch's spirit is the essence, inner motivation, and soul. Spirit is the impetus behind your magickal workings and the power force of your inner witch. A dampened, unhealthy spirit can convolute energy by placing too much emphasis on the low-brow drives of the ego over the higher-power drives of our authentic soul. The closer one comes to healing the spirit, the more pure and well intentioned the magickal workings. A healed spirit is also infectious and has a positive effect on our family, friends, and communities. After all, healed people heal others. Use these spells and rituals to root out any unhealthy ego-driven forces and embrace an inspired, compassionate, fearless you.

LOVE OPENING BURN AND BATHE

PURPOSE OF SPELL: This spell is meant to release you and heal you from past disappointment in love and renew your heart to the possibility of love.

SUGGESTED TIMING:
New moon

ITEMS NEEDED:

- Wooden spoon
- Mixing bowl
- Mason jar
- 2 candles
- Lighter
- Scrap of paper
- Black ink

ITEMS CONT.

- Small bowl
- Bathtub
- Bath mixture:
  1 cup Epsom salt,
  1 cup baking soda,
  1 teaspoon coconut oil

MAGICKAL INGREDIENTS:

- 8 drops frankincense oil
- 8 drops lavender oil

SPELLWORK

✦ Create a potion by adding the oils to the bath mixture in a mixing bowl. Stir the oils thoroughly into the bath mixture using the wooden spoon. Use half of this potion for a ritual love bath now and store the other half in the mason jar for use during the full moon in 2 weeks.

✦ Run your bathwater to desired temperature, adding in your potion once you plug the drain.

CONTINUED >>>

✦ Light two candles on your bathroom sink. One candle represents your future, and the other candle represents your past. Fill the small bowl with bathwater and place it between the candles. Write something symbolic of the past on the piece of paper—perhaps an ex-lover's name.

✦ Burn the paper with your lighter and chant:

> *"Goodbye disappointment, so long pain,*
> *I release you from my memory, I have only love to gain."*

✦ Drop the burning paper into the small bowl of bathwater and blow out the past candle.

✦ Get in the bath and submerse yourself in the warm, healing water. Notice your single candle burning with future positivity. Soak your body and your bones in the healing, renewing potion. When done, dry off and flush the bowl of burned paper and water down the toilet. Extinguish the remaining candle, knowing your future in love is looking bright. Repeat the cleansing bath with the other half of the potion in 2 weeks to complete the spell.

HONOR MOTHER NATURE

PURPOSE OF SPELL: This good morning ritual heals spiritual disconnect with Mother Nature and strengthens your alignment with natural cycles that power your craft.

SUGGESTED TIMING:
Dawn

ITEMS NEEDED:
• Spade and jar

MAGICKAL INGREDIENTS:
• Yourself

SPELLWORK

✦ Stand outside in a quiet, private location.

✦ Plant your feet firmly on the ground. Consider going barefoot if safe to do so.

✦ Face east. Center yourself. Appreciate your chosen location. On your next deep inhale, raise your arms overhead. With arms still raised, chant:

"I honor eastern air."

Exhale while lowering your arms.

CONTINUED >>>

✦ Turn to your right to face south. On your next deep inhale, **raise** your arms overhead. With arms raised, chant:

"I honor southern flame."

Exhale while lowering your arms.

✦ Continue this process for west:

"I honor western water."

✦ And north:

"I honor northern earth."

✦ When finished, bend down and scoop earth from where you **performed** the ceremony. Bring it home in a jar for your altar. **Ritual dirt** is great for drawing health into your life simply by **being** present in your home. Enjoy its magickal, healing energy.

✦ Discard after one moon cycle, and repeat the spell as needed.

STARGAZING MOON DANCER

PURPOSE OF SPELL: The purpose of this ritual is to heal any disconnect you feel with the universe and to connect with divine healing using the power of the cosmos.

SUGGESTED TIMING:
Full moon or eve of a major sabbat

ITEMS NEEDED:
- Bowl of water
- Bowl of salt
- Bell or chime

ITEMS CONT.
- Athame
- Journal or small piece of paper and pen

MAGICKAL INGREDIENTS:
- 1 amethyst crystal
- 1 clear quartz crystal

SPELLWORK

✦ Set your outdoor sacred space by placing the water to the west, the salt to the north, the bell to the east, and the athame to the south. These represent the elements of water, earth, air, and fire, respectively.

✦ Stand in the center of the four elements. Use your five senses to connect with nature. What does the air smell like? Is there a taste of moisture in the air? Do you hear a breeze rustling the trees? Feel the ground you are standing on. Finally, look up to the stars in the night sky.

CONTINUED >>>

✦ While looking up, raise your arms to the sky as if touching the stars. Wave your arms back and forth. Allow the motion to continue down your arms and into your head and torso. Start swaying your hips and maybe pirouette a bit on one leg. Dance to the music of the night sky. Dance to celebrate your place in the cosmos. Dance to accept divine presence into your life.

✦ When tired, sit and rest in the center of your four elements. Hold your amethyst and clear quartz near. Take your journal or piece of paper, and return your eyes to the night sky above you. Draw the position of the stars and the moon as you see them. Don't worry about accuracy or artistic talent. Focus on transcribing the moment as you are experiencing it, in the language of the stars. Refer to this magickal drawing and this magickal night when you need to remember your blessed, special place among the stars and to heal any recurring disconnect.

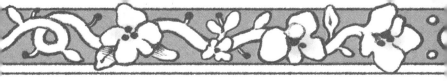

THE SEERS ROAD OPENING POTION

PURPOSE OF SPELL: Use this potion to enhance your spirit's receptivity to psychic messages and visions about your life path. Heal any sense of indirection or confusion you may have about your life's purpose and future by applying this potion to your magickal workings.

SUGGESTED TIMING:
Full moon

ITEMS NEEDED:

- Small saucepan
- 2 tablespoons olive oil
- Cheesecloth
- Small jar

MAGICKAL INGREDIENTS:

- 3 sprigs of rosemary
- 3 sprigs of thyme
- 3 sage leaves
- ¼ cup dried lavender
- 3 drops cedarwood essential oil

SPELLWORK

✦ Heat oil in the saucepan over medium heat until shimmery and viscous.

✦ Stir in the rosemary, thyme, sage, and lavender, adding more oil if needed to fully cover the herbs. Simmer on low for 5 to 10 minutes. Stir occasionally.

✦ Remove from heat and let sit for another 3 to 5 minutes.

✦ Strain the cooling mixture through the cheesecloth and into the jar.

CONTINUED >>>

✦ Discard the leftover herbs outside as an offering to Mother Earth.

✦ Add the cedar oil to the jar.

✦ Shake the potion well, repeating:

> *"Soothsayers and sibyls, oracles and prophets*
> *Lend me your talents, show me my way.*
> *By herbs and by oil, I divine my life purpose*
> *Open my road, 'til my last dying day."*

✦ Charge the potion under full moonlight. Use for clarity as needed by dabbing onto your third eye, temples, or heart. Alternatively, use the potion in spellwork to anoint candles for help making life decisions or starting new ventures.

AN OPEN BOOK

PURPOSE OF SPELL: This spell helps heal any disconnect in your intuition and weakness in your psychic abilities. It uses the magick of bibliomancy, or divination using books, to help you receive guidance from the divine. By invoking your intuition and intuitive tools, you are able to receive divine messages through written words and heal from divine disconnect.

SUGGESTED TIMING:
Waxing moon, full moon

ITEMS NEEDED:

- A favorite book or a book that has meaning to your soul. Perhaps it is a novel that changed your life, a book of poems that inspire, or a spiritual text like the Torah or Bible. The more familiar, connected, and invested in the text you are the better.

ITEMS CONT.

- Essential oil diffuser
- ½ cup salt

MAGICKAL INGREDIENTS:

- 3 amethyst crystals
- 3 sodalite crystals
- 3 clear quartz crystals
- Essential oil blend:
  4 drops lavender,
  3 drops bergamot

SPELLWORK

✦ Sit on the floor in a quiet, comfortable location with your chosen book.

✦ Turn on your diffuser containing your essential oil blend nearby.

CONTINUED >>>

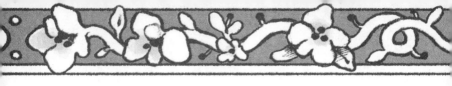

✦ Create a circle around yourself with a thin line of salt. Set points of amethyst, sodalite, and clear quartz along the salt to create a protective grid of intuitive energy.

✦ Hold the book in your hands and press it to your forehead, letting the energy of the book meld with your mind for a minute or so. Breathe deeply and evenly the entire time.

✦ As you press the book to your body, ask spirit to speak to you through the medium of your book.

✦ Chant three times:

> *"Spirit divine, hear my plea,*
> *Use this book to message me*
> *Words of guidance and words of light*
> *I receive your meaning clear and bright."*

✦ At the end of the third chant, allow the book to fall open in your lap. Instantly place your finger where it is drawn to on the page. Read the passage spirit has chosen for you to see. Consider its meaning. Contemplate the passage's place in the book at large. Then think about the message in the context of the current events of your life. How can you apply this message? Remember, spirit wants to help you, so try to formulate advice for yourself out of the passage. Trust that this process is healing your intuition, and trust spirit to speak the truth you need to hear.

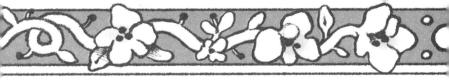

CHARMED AND ARMED

PURPOSE OF SPELL: This charm draws magickal protection to your spirit using the magick of defensive crystals, herbs, and spices. Heal chinks in your spiritual armor with this sachet charm.

SUGGESTED TIMING:
Waxing moon, full moon

ITEMS NEEDED:

- Lighter
- Small muslin bag or cloth square

MAGICKAL INGREDIENTS:

- Bundle of dried sage
- 3 bay leaves
- 1 tablespoon dried parsley
- 1 tablespoon ground sage
- 1 fluorite crystal
- 1 clear quartz crystal

SPELLWORK

✦ Lay out all ingredients on your altar separately.

✦ Light the dried sage and wave the smoke over all the ingredients and yourself to cleanse any attached negative energies.

✦ Next, enchant these ingredients for protection. Lightly lay your hands on the items and incant:

> *"I invoke protection from these crystals and herbs*
> *Keep me from harm and tumultuous curves.*
> *Hold me in safety, free of doubt, harm, and fear*
> *I am protected from danger when this charm is near."*

CONTINUED >>>

✦ Put all blessed ingredients into the bag or tie them up together in the cloth square. Wear on your person, keep in a pocket or purse, or display on your altar. Grasp the sachet for protective energy whenever you feel the need to heal your spiritual protection. Recharge under the full moon each month.

THE HEALING POWER OF WITCHCRAFT

SMOKE DIVINATION PRAXIS

PURPOSE OF SPELL: Change is hard to accept. As creatures of habit, we often feel out of sorts, confused, or even angry when changes occur. Heal your negative, stress-filled responses to change through the praxis of smoke divination magick.

SUGGESTED TIMING:
Waning moon, new moon

ITEMS NEEDED:
- Candle
- Lighter
- Small bowl of water

ITEMS CONT.
- Athame
- Bell

MAGICKAL INGREDIENTS:
- 1 jasper crystal
- 1 drop lavender oil

SPELLWORK

✦ Set your candle in the center of your altar and anoint it with the lavender oil. Surround your candle with the power of the four directions by placing the crystal to the north of the candle, the athame to the south of the candle, the small bowl of water to the west, and the bell to the east.

✦ Light the candle. Stare intently at the dancing flame. Watch as it dips and moves to the rhythm of the worldly energy within and without. Meditate on the change happening in your life. Think about how it came to be, and think about how you are

CONTINUED >>>

currently handling the change. Ask yourself if you are responding in the healthiest way or if adjustments need to be made. Finally, call on spirit for divine guidance with the change through the power of smoke.

✦ When ready, blow out your candle. Follow the direction of the smoke with your eyes. Did it head north toward your crystal? Or a different direction? Here is what the direction of the smoke and type of smoke means to aid you in understanding, accepting, and healing from change:

SMOKE RISES STRAIGHT UP: Spirit advises nothing is to be done. Simply release and lean into the change.

SMOKE RISES TO THE NORTH: This change will require your leadership and confidence; it's time to rise to the challenge and step into your power.

SMOKE RISES TO THE SOUTH: This change will likely be difficult and chaotic; allow yourself grace with its challenges.

SMOKE RISES TO THE EAST: This change brings wonderful new beginnings; look for opportunities.

SMOKE RISES TO THE WEST: This change closes a chapter in your life; let that chapter go.

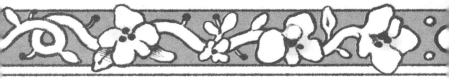

ABUNDANT SMOKE: Hurry to act on the change.

THIN, WISPY SMOKE: Take your time processing the change.

✦ By intentionally exploring your response to change with this divination method, you are healing from, and working through, the change in your life.

SPIRIT INSPIRATION RITUAL

PURPOSE OF SPELL: Conjure inspiration for your spirit by using air magick power of meaningful, spoken words to uplift and heal you from a spiritual rut.

SUGGESTED TIMING:
This prayer ritual is invoked at dawn, signifying new beginnings.

ITEMS NEEDED:

- Candle
- Lighter
- Pen and paper

MAGICKAL INGREDIENTS:

- 1 citrine crystal
- 1 carnelian crystal

SPELLWORK

✦ On the night before performing this ritual, sit at your desk and light a candle to draw sparks of inspiration to you. Write a list of 12 things that inspire your soul. Don't be afraid to dig deep and get creative. These can be physical inspirations like good books, your favorite artist, flowers, or your children. These may also be intangible inspirations such as laughter, wind in the trees, the sound of the ocean crashing, or the energy of your crystals.

✦ Once you have solidified your list, write one sentence next to each item that describes the quality of the item that most inspires you. For example, "Mary Cassatt inspires my spirit's love of beauty and my care for my children as their mother." Or, "The sound of the ocean inspires my spirit to find its rhythm."

✦ When finished, place the crystals on your page overnight to charge the words.

✦ The next morning, stand firmly in a meaningful outdoor location, list in one hand, crystals in the other.

✦ Let the power of earth and air combine in your flowing words. Your spirit heals as you read your list aloud as a prayer to Mother Nature. To remind you of this healing moment, select a rock from the ground where you are standing and bring it home to your altar as a keepsake of this healing renewal.

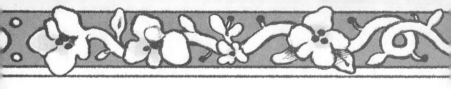

GUILT BE GONE

PURPOSE OF SPELL: Guilt is a heavy burden, especially when we are truly sorry or when we feel guilty for things beyond our control. Heal your spirit from the burden of guilt by engaging the lightness of air magick.

SUGGESTED TIMING:
Waning moon, new moon; select a clear, dry night so as not to damage the cloth.

ITEMS NEEDED:
- 1 scarf, blanket, or sweatshirt you use often and that comforts you.
- A safe outdoor location to hang the cloth from, such as a clothesline, tree branch, balcony, porch, or open window.

ITEMS CONT.
- Small bowl

MAGICKAL INGREDIENTS:
- Sodalite crystals
- Smoky quartz crystals

SPELLWORK

✦ After sunset, hang your special cloth or piece of clothing outside.

✦ Tie the crystals into the cloth or place them just beneath the cloth in a bowl.

✦ Stand with your arms raised out to the cloth, and call on the power of air by incanting:

"Wind blow fierce or wind blow gently
North or south blow relief aplenty
East and west cleanse my burdened soul
Power of air, please make me whole."

✦ Leave the cloth outside overnight, allowing the crystals, night air, and moonlight to cleanse and renew.

✦ Bring the cloth and crystals inside in the morning and allow any dew to dry. Wrap your cloth around you when you need to ease guilt from your mind. The magickally charged cloth will help remove the burden and heal you with magickal comfort.

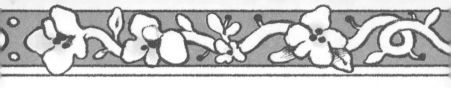

LITTLE ALTAR OF ALIGNMENT

PURPOSE OF SPELL: Your spirit is healed through the alignment of your mind and body. When your mind and body are aligned, the spirit flows naturally. This spell creates a mini ritual altar of mind/body alignment that makes for a healthy, flourishing spirit.

SUGGESTED TIMING:
As needed

ITEMS NEEDED:
- Windowsill space or a small table next to a sunny window

MAGICKAL INGREDIENTS:
- Chakra-opening stones:
  Clear quartz: Crown chakra
  Amethyst: Third-eye chakra
  Sodalite: Throat chakra
  Green aventurine:
    Heart chakra
  Citrine: Solar plexus
  Carnelian: Sacral chakra
  Jasper: Root chakra

SPELLWORK

✦ Oftentimes our body does not feel aligned with what our mind wants. Our head is telling us one thing while our gut is telling us another. We feel confused about what actions to take next. This confusion takes the wind out of our sails and deflates the spirit. To help, use the power of crystals to open your seven chakras, or bodily energy centers, and align your thoughts with your actions.

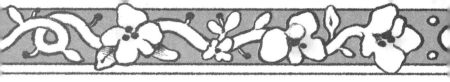

✦ Begin by placing the clear quartz on the top of your head. Incant:

"Power of quartz, open for me, the depths of my spirituality."

Set the quartz on the windowsill.

✦ Place the amethyst on your forehead. Incant:

"Power of amethyst, open for me, allow my third eye to see."

Set the amethyst next to the quartz on the windowsill.

✦ Place the sodalite on your throat. Incant:

"Power of sodalite, open for me,
The ability to speak the truth freely."

Set the sodalite next to the amethyst on the windowsill.

✦ Place the green aventurine on your heart. Incant:

"Power of aventurine, open for me,
Fill my heart with joy and glee."

Set the aventurine next to the sodalite on the windowsill.

✦ Place the citrine on your abdomen. Incant:

"Power of citrine, open for me, willpower and intentionality."

Set the citrine next to the aventurine on the windowsill.

✦ Place the carnelian on your pelvis. Incant:

"Power of carnelian, open for me, imagination and creativity."

Set the carnelian next to the citrine on the windowsill.

✦ Finally, place the jasper on your lower back. Incant:

"Power of jasper, open for me, a sense of home and security."

Set the jasper next to the carnelian on your windowsill.

✦ Take in the beauty of the sunlight dancing on your mini altar of openness and alignment. Let this image and energy totally synthesize your mind and body to produce a healed, flourishing spirit.

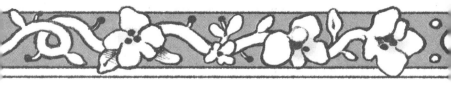

FORGIVING FOOT SOAK

PURPOSE OF SPELL: Your spirit is healed through forgiveness. Use this magickal foot soak to summon forgiveness for those who have wronged you. Often anger is justified and warranted, even righteous. For the sake of our own precious spiritual energy, though, it is productive to eventually try to forgive at some point. Even if the person does not deserve forgiveness, think of it as a release. This person is no longer allowed to trigger you, as you have moved on in clarity and in compassion for your spirit.

SUGGESTED TIMING:
Waning moon, new moon

ITEMS NEEDED:
- Large, heat-safe bowl
- Boiling water

MAGICKAL INGREDIENTS:
- 1 tablespoon cinnamon powder
- 2 tablespoons chamomile
- 1 tablespoon lavender
- 1 amethyst crystal
- 1 smoky quartz crystal

SPELLWORK

✦ Place the bowl on the floor next to a chair. Add the cinnamon, herbs, and crystals to the bowl.

✦ Pour boiling water over the mixture and incant:

> *"Fiery anger, hot like this boiling water,*
> *Soak my calming rocks and spices,*
> *And so this anger begins to falter."*

CONTINUED >>>

◆ Lean down and inhale the calming energy of the heat-activated spices and herbs for a few moments.

◆ While the water cools a bit, stand straight with your bare feet on the ground. As you stand tall and proud, push all the anger energy you are holding on to from the top of your head down through your torso, down your legs, and into your feet. Feel the anger collect heavily in your feet. Feel the burden of the painful outrage. Let it hurt.

◆ Now have a seat. Move your feet into the herbal water, carefully testing first that it is safe to do so. Immerse your feet fully in the healing herbs. Massage your feet on the crystals. Imagine all the dark, fiery rage slowly being drawn out of your feet by the magickal water. Begin to feel peace. Begin to feel wholeness. Know you are healing from this difficult experience. Discard the cooled water outside in a storm drain or river to let forgiveness flow freely, emanating far and wide.

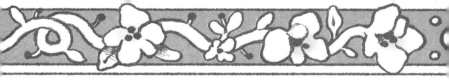

LEAVES OF HOPE

PURPOSE OF SPELL: Your spirit suffers from lack of hope or belief in your dreams. This spell heals this doubt and releases your heart's greatest hopes and desires out into the universe for fulfillment using the power of fire and bay leaf.

SUGGESTED TIMING:
New moon

ITEMS NEEDED:

- Cauldron filled with 2 inches of salt
- Long lighter

MAGICKAL INGREDIENTS:

- 4 whole, dried bay leaves

SPELLWORK

✦ Think of four wishes or hopes you would like the new moon to bless. Assign a wish to each bay leaf by holding each leaf to your lips as you whisper the wish to it.

✦ Arrange each leaf in the salt with one end in the salt and the other sticking straight up. Place them in north, south, east, and west locations.

CONTINUED >>>

✦ When you are ready, burn each bay leaf down to the salt, one at a time. (This is why I recommend a long lighter, as you may have to hold the flame on each leaf as it burns to keep it going.) This spell is about inertia, so we want that bay leaf in ashes to complete the wish. Start by burning the northern wish and move clockwise through the western wish. Take your time and feel the power of each intention.

✦ As you burn each leaf, imagine yourself living the best outcome of each wish and heal your doubts.

✦ Chant:

"Hail Goddess, blessed be, grant my hopes and wishes unto me!"

✦ Discard the ashes outside to seal the spell with Mother Nature and jump-start the process of healing your spirit with this renewal of your hopes and dreams.

COURAGE COCKTAIL

PURPOSE OF SPELL: Your spirit is hurting when you cannot summon confidence and courage. Create an altar display that calls on the power of oils, herbs, and crystals to bolster confidence and courage and heal your spirit's insecurities.

SUGGESTED TIMING:
Waxing moon, full moon

ITEMS NEEDED:

- Martini glass, margarita glass, or wineglass
- Salt

MAGICKAL INGREDIENTS:

- 3 bay leaves
- 3 sprigs of thyme
- 3 whole sage leaves
- Citrine crystals
- Tourmaline crystals
- Essential oil blend:
  3 drops orange,
  3 drops cedar,
  3 drops frankincense

SPELLWORK

✦ Fill the bottom third of your selected glassware with salt. Sprinkle the essential oil drops over the salt.

✦ Lay the bay leaves and sage flat over the oiled salt.

✦ Place the crystals on top of the leaves. Feel free to add a lot of crystals here if you have them to make a beautiful arrangement.

CONTINUED >>>

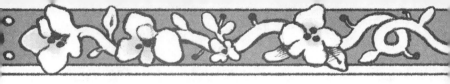

✦ Garnish the glass with the thyme.

✦ Set the glass to charge overnight by the light of the waxing/ full moon. Keep this courage cocktail on your altar for up to 3 days and nights to inspire your spirit with confidence and heal timidity.

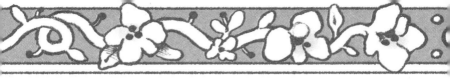

ELEMENTAL RESOLVE

PURPOSE OF SPELL: As a healing warrior for yourself and others, your spirit will encounter a lot of negative energy and can, at times, feel deflated. Use this spell to refresh and renew your spirit from these negative energies.

SUGGESTED TIMING:
New moon

ITEMS NEEDED:

- Bowl of warm water, preferably warmed moon water elixir from Healing Moon Water Elixir (see page 66).
- Essential oil diffuser

MAGICKAL INGREDIENTS:

- 1 rose quartz crystal
- 1 citrine crystal
- Bergamot oil or lavender oil for your diffuser (choose the scent you most prefer)

SPELLWORK

✦ Turn on your diffuser with your chosen oil.

✦ Sit comfortably in front of your altar, holding one stone in each fist.

✦ When ready, press the crystals to your face and chant:

"Power of air, cleanse my vision and my voice."

CONTINUED >>>

✦ Press the crystals to your heart and chant:

"Power of earth, strengthen my heart and my hopes."

✦ Next, press the crystals to your pelvic area and chant:

"Power of fire, inspire compassion and creativity."

✦ Finally, place your fists into the bowl of warm water. Release your crystals into the bowl of water, leaving your hands in the water. Chant:

"Power of water, renew self-worth and renew my soul."

✦ Remove your hands, allowing them to air dry on your lap as you continue to sit and breathe slowly, leaning into the pulsating self-love energy you just created. Match your deep breaths to this loving energy flow. By the time your hands are dry, the spell is sealed. You will continue on with your day with a healed spirit, in resolve born anew.

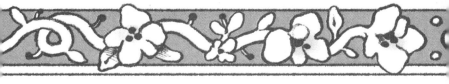

THE RIPPLE EFFECT OF TRUTH

PURPOSE OF SPELL: Now that you are well on your way to healing your body, mind, and spirit, it is time to use your healed outlook to embrace healing righteousness. It is time to find your voice and the courage to speak truth to power. You have spent so much time and energy learning your truth, it is time to aid others by sharing your knowledge and your wisdom. This spell prepares you and strengthens your spirit for important healing work ahead that you will direct to your communities and the world.

SUGGESTED TIMING:
Full moon

ITEMS NEEDED:
- Bowl filled with warm water placed on your altar
- Bottle with lid

MAGICKAL INGREDIENTS:
- Sprigs of thyme
- Sprigs of mint
- 3 citrine crystals
- 3 sodalite crystals
- 1 clear quartz crystal

SPELLWORK

✦ Begin by circling your bowl with alternating citrine and sodalite stones. Fill in the gaps of the crystal circle with a wreath of strengthening sprigs of thyme and inspiring, truth-filled mint leaves. Feel the energies of the stones and herbs envelop and penetrate your bowl of warm water from the outside in. Consider how effective the magickal energy can be on

CONTINUED >>>

the water, even if they are not in direct contact. So is the effect of your power to help others.

✦ When ready, hold the clear quartz stone a few inches above the center of the water bowl. Incant:

> *"Stone of balance and clarity,*
> *Amplify my voice and my energy.*
> *Ripple my healing intentions far and wide*
> *I will speak my healing truth, I will no longer hide."*

✦ Drop the stone into the water. Watch the splash and ripple effect closely. Let the waves of energy wash over you, strengthening you, until the water stills and the spell seals.

✦ Bottle the water and add a few drops to your morning tea, coffee, or shake to infuse your throat and solar plexus with the power of truth. Your spirit will remain strong for the healing work ahead of you with this magickal Ripple Water.

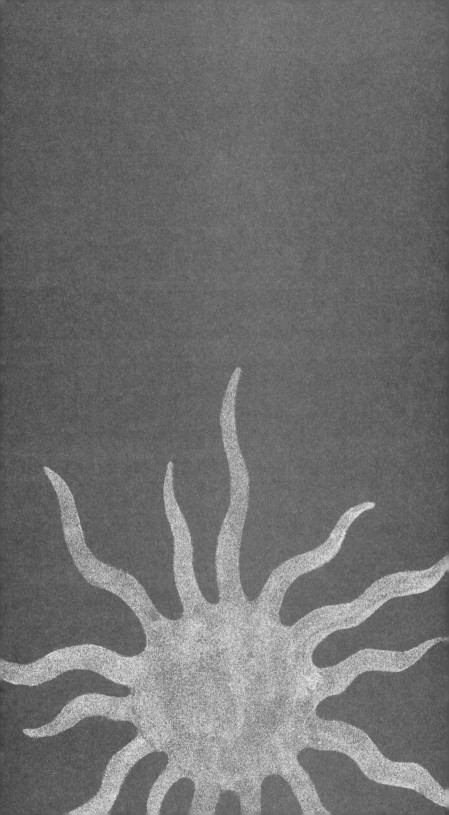

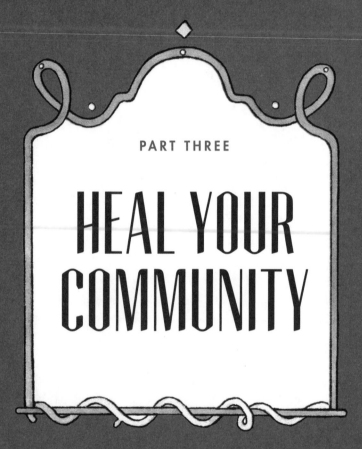

PART THREE

HEAL YOUR COMMUNITY

A WITCH IS CALLED TO ACTION BY THE NATURE of our healing powers. We are a beacon of light and hope to others, and we use our powers to make positive change. As we heal ourselves, we come to understand our call as witches is also to help and heal others. Furthermore, we know when others heal, they too positively impact their loved ones and communities. The chain reaction of healing light is powerful indeed. The spells that follow are intended to direct your inner healing light outward for the exponential benefit of all.

HEAL YOUR FRIENDS AND FAMILY

We begin to turn our magick outward to our friends and family in order to heal their troubles through sympathy magick. Sympathy magick is magick we perform on behalf of our loved ones who may be struggling to heal physically, mentally, or spiritually. In the spells and rituals that follow, you will find ways to direct your healing energies to help make positive changes in the lives of those people you care about.

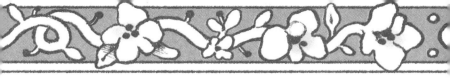

HEALING POPPET

PURPOSE OF SPELL: This spell uses the power of poppets (small dolls or trinkets that represent another person) to send caring, healing vibes to friends and family afflicted with illness.

SUGGESTED TIMING:
New moon

ITEMS NEEDED:

- Lighter
- Poppet
- Bowl large enough to fit the poppet

MAGICKAL INGREDIENTS:

- 1 tablespoon dried sage or a dried sage bundle
- 1 cup lavender
- ¼ teaspoon black pepper
- Rose quartz crystals
- Sodalite crystals
- Fluorite crystals
- 3 drops tea tree oil

SPELLWORK

✦ Light the sage and let it smoke. Pass the poppet through the smoke to cleanse it of any unwanted energies that may interfere with the spell.

✦ Next, anoint the poppet with three drops of tea tree oil, speaking the name of the person you mean to heal as you work.

✦ Mix the lavender and black pepper in the bowl. Gently lay the poppet in the bowl, and seal the poppet to the bowl of healing magick with a kiss.

CONTINUED >>>

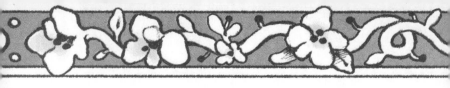

✦ Surround the poppet with rose quartz, sodalite, and fluorite crystals.

✦ Keep the resting poppet bowl in a comfortable location in your home. Consider placing the poppet on your dresser, among house plants, near a sunny window, or on your mantel.

✦ Care for the poppet daily by whispering healing messages and words of love to it. Continue this healing magick every day until the night of the full moon, when the spell will be complete.

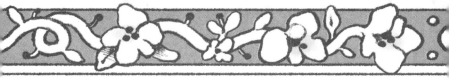

SWEET SUTURES SACHET

PURPOSE OF SPELL: This spell uses the power of healing herbs and crystals to help your friends and family recover from surgery.

SUGGESTED TIMING:
As needed

ITEMS NEEDED:
- Small muslin or cloth bag
- Needle and thread
- Pen with black ink

MAGICKAL INGREDIENTS:
- 3 whole, dry bay leaves
- 3 sprigs of thyme
- 1 black tourmaline crystal
- 1 green aventurine crystal

SPELLWORK

✦ Using the pen with black ink, write the name of the person recovering from surgery on each of the three bay leaves. Place the bay leaves in the bag. Add the thyme and crystals to the bag.

✦ Lay your hands over the contents of the bag and incant:

> *"Bay leaf three, thyme leaf three,*
> *Work your healing strength for me.*
> *By stone of green and stone of black,*
> *Disperse their pain and send it back."*

✦ Suture the bag closed with needle and thread, pouring loving, binding healing into each stitch as you sew. Give the bag to your patient for healing energy or keep it close to a picture of the person in recovery.

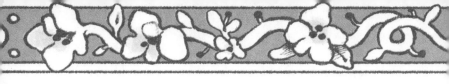

CLOVE PENTAGRAM

PURPOSE OF SPELL: Create this clove pentagram in salt to combat tough times for your loved one and disperse negative energies.

SUGGESTED TIMING:
New moon

ITEMS NEEDED:
- Plate or shallow bowl
- 1 cup salt

MAGICKAL INGREDIENTS:
- 1 cup whole cloves
- 1 green aventurine crystal

SPELLWORK

✦ Spread the salt evenly over the plate or shallow bowl. Feel free to add more if needed for the size plate you are using. You want a cushy base of salt, not just a dusting.

✦ Create a pentagram using the whole cloves on top of the salt. Place each clove, one by one, end to end, to create the outline of the pentagram. Notice how tedious, and lengthy, and frustrating the process can be. Pour those emotions into your creation, shifting them away from your loved ones who are also experiencing them.

✦ Seal the creation by placing abundance-drawing green aventurine in the center of the pentagram. Leave this pentagram on your altar until the full moon, when the spell to help your loved ones through tough times will be complete.

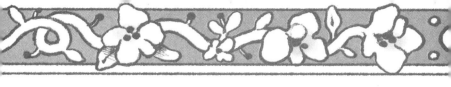

ROSEMARY LOVE BINDING

PURPOSE OF SPELL: This ritual is performed to help those in committed relationships through rough patches and to heal their love for each other.

SUGGESTED TIMING:
Start 7 days prior to the night of the full moon.

ITEMS NEEDED:
- A photograph of the couple, folded in half so their faces touch
- String or twine

MAGICKAL INGREDIENTS:
- 7 sprigs of rosemary
- 7 drops cedar oil to return love or 7 drops ylang-ylang oil to return passion

SPELLWORK

✦ Tie the string around the picture, leaving a little bit of give. Leave the folded picture on your altar.

✦ Each night, anoint one sprig of rosemary with one drop of oil. Slide the anointed sprig of rosemary under the string but on top of the folded photograph.

CONTINUED >>>

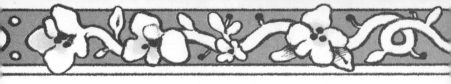

✦ Incant:

"Rosemary of strengthened love, rosemary of fidelity,
Rosemary of true connection, rosemary of longevity.
Anointed in oil to return love to this couple,
Cure their rough patch and bring love strong and supple."

✦ Repeat every night until the full moon, when your photograph will have seven sprigs of love-healing rosemary tied on top of it. On the night of the full moon, burn the picture. Scatter the ashes of the picture and the rosemary outside under the light of the full moon to seal the spell and reconcile the couple's love and passion.

THE HEALING POWER OF WITCHCRAFT

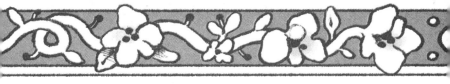

CALMING WATERS

PURPOSE OF SPELL: Use this water-bowl spell to ease the anxieties of your loved ones and send their minds off to calm waters.

SUGGESTED TIMING:
Waning moon

ITEMS NEEDED:
- Heat-safe bowl
- Boiling water
- Athame

MAGICKAL INGREDIENTS:
- 1 teaspoon allspice
- 1 teaspoon ground clove
- ½ cup star anise

SPELLWORK

✦ Add all spices to the heat-safe bowl. Charge them by drawing a spiral with your athame, starting at the center and circling outward to send the magick toward your loved ones.

✦ Pour the boiling water over the spices and fill the bowl.

✦ As the steam rises, incant three times:

"Rise steam of calm, rise wave of peace
Healing vibes and tranquility are released."

✦ Let the water cool as the spell's energy is sent to your loved ones. Discard the water outside to return any remaining healing energy to the earth.

DUMB SUPPER FOR THE GRIEVING

PURPOSE OF SPELL: This ritual provides space to sit with our grief after the passing of a loved one in order to heal our hurting hearts and help lift the weight of grief.

SUGGESTED TIMING:

A Dumb Supper is traditionally hosted at Samhain to honor our deceased loved ones but may be performed on the first full moon after the passing of a loved one as well.

ITEMS NEEDED:

- Favorite meal of the deceased
- An extra, empty place setting at your dinner table for the deceased

ITEMS CONT.

- Bowl for herb and crystal centerpiece
- 2 candles
- Lighter

MAGICKAL INGREDIENTS:

- Stalks of parsley, fresh or dried
- 3 heads of garlic, unpeeled
- Smoky quartz crystals
- Black tourmaline crystals
- Clear quartz crystals

SPELLWORK

✦ Place the parsley in the center of the bowl. Arrange the three heads of garlic and crystals around and on top of the parsley.

✦ Place a candle on either side of this centerpiece, one to signify this world and one to signify the world beyond.

✦ Light the candles and incant:

"In this world and in the beyond, we dine tonight in silent bond."

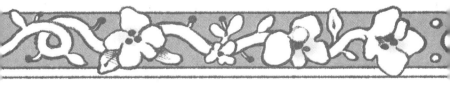

✦ Continue in complete silence. The silence you observe together is in reverence for the empty place. Use this silent time to think privately of fond memories of the deceased. You may cry or laugh a bit. Let your grief be your guide.

✦ In silence, serve the meal you have cooked to yourself (and others if you have invited guests) and also to the empty space. Eat together in silence. When finished, blow out the candles. Clear the table of everything in silence, leaving only the "dumb supper" of the deceased, the magick centerpiece, and the extinguished candles. Cover the supper in saran wrap if you desire.

✦ Leave the supper out overnight. In the morning, discard the supper and with it the weight of your grief. Know your love has reached across worlds and nourished your departed loved one. They, in turn, nourish you right back. Always.

HEART OF THE EARTH

PURPOSE OF SPELL: This spell helps ensure a long life by clearing and healing the body of any energy that dampens longevity.

SUGGESTED TIMING:
Full moon

ITEMS NEEDED:

- 1 whole apple
- Athame
- String

MAGICKAL INGREDIENTS:

- 3 sprigs of parsley
- ¼ teaspoon cinnamon

SPELLWORK

✦ Lightly etch the initials of the person this spell is intended for on the face of the apple.

✦ Incant:

> *"By fruit of autumn, I proclaim*
> *The longest life for whom I have named*
> *Cinnamon brings good luck in well-being*
> *Parsley wards negative energy and feeling."*

✦ Cut the apple in half widthwise with your athame to reveal the magickal five-pointed star inside.

✦ Sprinkle cinnamon on one half of the apple's flesh.

o   THE HEALING POWER OF WITCHCRAFT

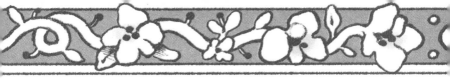

✦ Tie the three sprigs of parsley to the other half of the apple with the string.

✦ Eat the apple half with cinnamon. You may also offer it to the person you are performing the spell for if they would like to partake. The consumption of the magick into our bodily systems is powerful healing.

✦ Bury the other half of the apple with parsley attached outside. This will return all bad energies the person may be carrying to the earth for cleansing and rejuvenation.

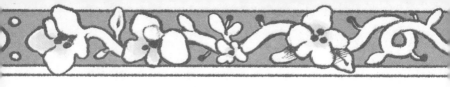

CRYSTAL ENERGY SUNDIAL

PURPOSE OF SPELL: This ritual will combat and heal the lethargic effects of the day-to-day grind on your friends and family. By harnessing the power of the sun through this crystal grid, you will keep lively, dynamic, and passionate vibes inspiring your loved one all day long.

SUGGESTED TIMING:
As needed

ITEMS NEEDED:
- Secure outdoor location under the shining sun
- Cutting board or plate

MAGICKAL INGREDIENTS:
- 4 clear quartz crystals
- 4 citrine crystals
- 4 carnelian crystals
- 4 drops eucalyptus oil

SPELLWORK

✦ Put four drops of eucalyptus oil in the center of your board or plate. As you pour each drop, say the name of the person you are helping with this spell.

✦ Next, place the crystals in a circle around the eucalyptus drops in the likeness of a clock.

Place the clear quartz on the 12, 3, 6, and 9 spots.

Place the citrine on the 1, 4, 7, and 10 spots.

Place the carnelian on the 2, 5, 8, and 11 spots.

✦ Leave the grid out until sunset to draw down the energy of the sun and disperse it to energize your loved one.

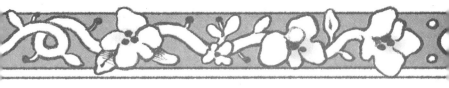

MIRROR, MIRROR, MENTAL HEALTH

PURPOSE OF SPELL: This spell gives a healing boost of love and light to those in your life struggling with mental health.

SUGGESTED TIMING:
After sunset, as needed

ITEMS NEEDED:

- Small mirror placed flat on your altar
- Candle
- Small bowl
- Lighter
- Cotton swab
- Small bowl of water

MAGICKAL INGREDIENTS:

- 4 chamomile sprigs
- Rose quartz crystals
- Jasper crystals
- Clear quartz crystals
- Essential oil blend:
  3 drops bergamot oil,
  3 drops orange oil

SPELLWORK

✦ Place your candle in the center of the mirror.

✦ Mix your oils in a small bowl with a cotton swab. Draw a heart with your oiled swab on the candle to charge it with loving vibes. Apply more oil on your swab to write the initials of the person you are healing on the mirror, just below the candle.

✦ Line the edges of the mirror with the crystals and chamomile to create a healing energy wall.

CONTINUED >>>

✦ Darken the room of all artificial light. Light the candle in the center of the mirror. Allow the flame to grow tall and strong under your watchful gaze. As the flame begins to melt the candle, feel the energy of love and healing release. Watch the flame dance in the mirror. Watch how this healing energy is now magnified by the mirror's infinite power.

✦ Direct the healing glow to the mental health of your target by incanting:

"Magick of earth and fire unite,
To pierce the lonely, darkened night.
Flame, rock, and herb combine, mental healing is inclined.
By the power of mirrored air, I send this healing magick there."

✦ Let the candle burn for as long as you feel is necessary for the healing energy to transfer. Usually 20 minutes to an hour of burn time is enough. Use your intuition to judge the needed length of burn.

✦ When ready to finish, incant:

"I leave this healing love in the mind of my friend,
Now with the power of water I bring their anguish to end."

✦ Extinguish the candle directly into the small bowl of healing water to seal the spell.

THE HEALING POWER OF WITCHCRAFT

STICKING TOGETHER

PURPOSE OF SPELL: This spell heals discord between friends and works to repair friendships.

SUGGESTED TIMING:
New moon

ITEMS NEEDED:

- One 12-inch stick foraged locally
- One 12-inch strand of string or ribbon to represent each person in the fight
- Athame

ITEMS CONT.

- Candle
- Lighter

MAGICKAL INGREDIENTS:

- Sodalite crystals
- Fluorite crystals
- Sweet orange oil (as much as needed)

SPELLWORK

✦ Use your athame to carve the initials of all friends involved in the discord into the wooden stick.

✦ Add one drop of orange oil to seal each name in friendship.

✦ Tie each string to the top of the stick, letting the majority of each string hang down alongside the stick. You will have a knot of multiple strings at the top of your stick.

CONTINUED >>>

✦ Light your candle. Allow the healing light to shine on the stick for a few moments as the wax begins to melt. Pick up your candle and tip it so the wax drips and melts over the string knots at the top of the stick. Let the wax harden.

✦ Next, braid and twist all strings about the sticks, entwining their energies together. Seal the ends of the string to the end of the stick with more wax from your candle. Extinguish the candle when done.

✦ Place the stick by a window alongside some sodalite and fluorite crystals. Allow the new moon to bless new beginnings of friendships healed by your magickal stick.

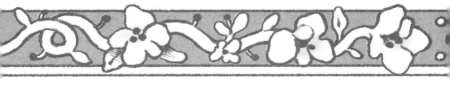

TO THYSELF BE TRUE

PURPOSE OF SPELL: Oftentimes our friends and family struggle to be accepted for their authentic identities. Perform this spell when your friend or family member needs to heal from the pressure to be something they are not and feel good about themselves as they are.

SUGGESTED TIMING:
New moon

ITEMS NEEDED:

- Round plate
- Candle
- Lighter

MAGICKAL INGREDIENTS:

- 1 cup dried lavender
- 7 sprigs of fresh thyme
- 1 clear quartz crystal
- 1 amethyst crystal
- 1 sodalite crystal
- 1 green aventurine crystal
- 1 citrine crystal
- 1 carnelian crystal
- 1 jasper crystal

SPELLWORK

✦ Set the candle in the middle of the plate. Spread the lavender out evenly on the plate around the candle.

✦ Wrap each stone in a sprig of thyme to amplify the strength of each crystal's properties. Create a circle around the candle, atop the lavender bed, with the seven stones wrapped in thyme.

CONTINUED >>>

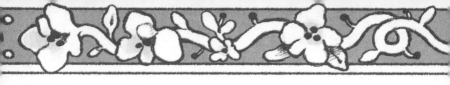

✦ When ready, light the candle and incant:

"The seven parts of [NAME] make them whole
From mind and body, to spirit and soul.

Quartz I bid thee power acceptance
Amethyst I bid thee power knowledge
Sodalite I bid thee power truth
Aventurine I bid thee power heart
Citrine I bid thee power self-esteem
Carnelian I bid thee power passion
Jasper I bid thee power sense of self

The seven parts of [NAME] make them whole
From mind and body to spirit and soul."

✦ Blow out the candle to send the energy of self-love and acceptance to its target.

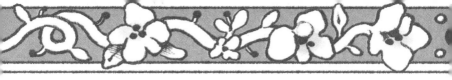

ACE AN OPPORTUNITY

PURPOSE OF SPELL: Whether it be a big job interview, an important test, a first date, or starting a new friendship, use this jar spell to heal your friends and family of the self-doubt that holds us back from truly embracing new opportunities.

SUGGESTED TIMING:
On the night before the big opportunity

ITEMS NEEDED:
- Medium-sized jar with the bottom third filled with salt
- Lighter
- Candle
- 1 tablespoon Epsom salt

ITEMS CONT.
- Small bowl

MAGICKAL INGREDIENTS:
- Citrine crystal stones or chips
- Essential oil blend:
  5 drops basil oil,
  5 drops bergamot oil,
  5 drops orange oil

SPELLWORK

✦ Mix the oils and Epsom salt together thoroughly in a small bowl. Spread the oil/Epsom salt mixture on top of the salt in the jar. Place the candle in the center of the jar, nestled in the salt.

✦ Line citrine around the inner rim of the jar.

✦ When ready, light the candle and loudly state the name of the person you are helping three times.

CONTINUED >>>

✦ Next, incant:

"Within salt of oil this flame is now lit
Amplified by the stone of courage and grit
Catch fire, take hold, burn bright, be bold
Stand firm, be proud, take up space, be loud.

All this helping magick
And this healing energy
All this I send to you
All this you will be."

✦ Say the name of the person again three times. Let the candle burn all the way down to the salt to seal the spell.

ADDICTION BIND AND FREEZE

PURPOSE OF SPELL: The road to recovery from addiction can be extremely difficult. Help your friends and family heal their harmful addictions with this spell to bind their impulses.

SUGGESTED TIMING:
Full moon

ITEMS NEEDED:

- Freezer-safe bowl/Tupperware with lid
- Small piece of bark or wood
- Athame
- Small bowl
- Small paintbrush or makeup brush

MAGICKAL INGREDIENTS:

- ½ cup lavender
- ½ cup thyme
- Carnelian crystals
- Essential oil blend:
  7 drops frankincense oil,
  7 drops cedar oil,
  3 drops peppermint oil

SPELLWORK

✦ Use your athame to etch the initials of the addicted person into the wood.

✦ Mix the oils together in a small bowl using a small paintbrush or makeup brush. Use the small paintbrush to coat the wood in the essential oils.

CONTINUED >>>

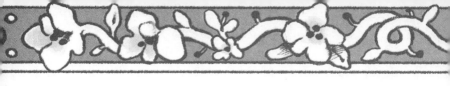

✦ As you paint, incant:

> *"Addiction be gone, impulse be free,*
> *Oils enlighten the way to recovery.*
> *As this magick works into the wood,*
> *So shall addiction be gone for good."*

✦ Set the oiled wood out to charge under the light of the full moon, surrounded by carnelian.

✦ In the morning, bring the wood inside. Place it in the freezer-safe bowl/Tupperware with the lavender and thyme. Fill the Tupperware with water and cover. Place it in the freezer until the new moon to seal the spell and bind the addiction.

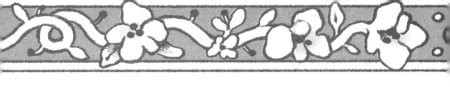

THE PAST DISPERSED, THE FUTURE UNCURSED

PURPOSE OF SPELL: Getting stuck in the past prevents us from embracing our true destiny. Heal the memories of your loved ones to encourage them to move on with their lives in confidence.

SUGGESTED TIMING:
Waning moon, new moon

ITEMS NEEDED:

- Piece of paper
- Pen with black ink
- Heat-safe bowl
- Hand towel
- Long lighter

MAGICKAL INGREDIENTS:

- ¼ cup lavender buds
- 1 bay leaf
- Dash of cayenne pepper

SPELLWORK

✦ On one side of the piece of paper, write all the things you can think of that are holding back this person from moving on with their lives. On the other side, write the person's name or initials. Draw a pentagram of protection over the person's name.

✦ Fill the bowl with boiling water and lavender buds. Drop the piece of paper into the boiling water and watch the ink dissolve.

CONTINUED >>>

Allow the water to cool as the buds soak up all the negativity from the words on the paper.

✦ Pick out the paper from the water and leave it to dry on a hand towel overnight. Discard the remaining water and lavender buds outside or down the toilet to ensure you are rid of the negative energies transferred.

✦ The next morning, place the now dried paper back in your empty heat-safe bowl. Add the bay leaf and cayenne pepper. Burn all three ingredients together into ash with a long lighter. Discard the ash outdoors or down the toilet to completely rid your loved one of that which is holding them back.

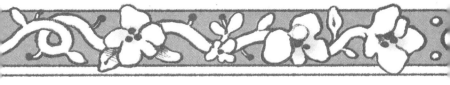

THE BOOK OF LOVE

PURPOSE OF SPELL: This spell is intended to infuse a constant energy of love and healing to those who matter most to you. By writing their names in a blessed location, you harness the lasting power of the written word. By allowing fresh herbs to dry in the pages, you are infusing herbal magick of love and healing in an eternal fashion.

SUGGESTED TIMING:
Full moon

ITEMS NEEDED:

- Blank notebook or your Book of Shadows
- Red ink pen
- Cotton swab

MAGICKAL INGREDIENTS:

- Sprig of fresh rosemary
- Basil essential oil

SPELLWORK

✦ By the light of the full moon, in red ink, write the name of every person you count worthy of your unconditional love and healing in your book.

✦ Add a drop or two of basil oil to your cotton swab. Seal each name by very lightly dabbing this oil of love and healing onto each name.

CONTINUED >>>

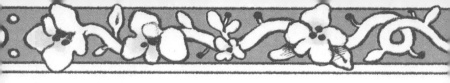

✦ As you dab, incant:

> *"The power of the written word seals my love for you*
> *The power of basil oil brings healing wishes true."*

✦ Finally, press the sprig of fresh rosemary onto this page of love for protection. Close the book tightly on the rosemary, adding more books on top for weight to press the rosemary alongside the oil and names within the pages of your book.

✦ Open your book to this page whenever a person written therein is suffering and in need of loving, healing energy.

HEAL GROUPS

As witchy individuals, we are part of many different groups in our lives. Perhaps we belong to a coven, but additionally most of us go to work, enjoy hobbies, and perform acts of service. Witches are members of online communities and digital social networks. We are members of neighborhoods and nations. Furthermore, as healers, we acknowledge our role in protecting disenfranchised groups, speaking truth to powerful groups, and leading the charge for social justice for all groups of people. No matter the identity of the groups we are part of, all groups contain massive amounts of energy that impact ourselves, other members of the group, and perhaps the world at large. In the spells that follow, you will learn how to harness group energy with the power of witchcraft to make positive, healing changes for groups and their communities in your life.

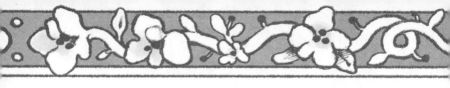

PROTECTIVE GROUP SIGIL

PURPOSE OF SPELL: Sigils are powerful symbols, created by the witch, to keep a constant stream of magick and intention flowing, even when our attention is elsewhere. Create a sigil based on the name of your group to use for group protection and a healing defense.

SUGGESTED TIMING:
New moon

ITEMS NEEDED:

- Paper
- Pen with black ink

MAGICKAL INGREDIENTS:

- Sprig of parsley
- 1 citrine crystal
- 1 carnelian crystal

SPELLWORK

✦ Write down the name of the group on the piece of paper. Discard all vowels and write the name again with just consonants. Notice how the consonants make interesting curves and angles in relation to each other.

✦ Stand with the paper on your altar and one crystal in each hand. Breathe in and out slowly while focusing on the consonants. Call on the energy of the citrine and carnelian to travel up your arms and infuse strength and creativity into your brain and heart. Feel your fingers and palms warm to the energy.

✦ As you start to feel the creative energy flowing stoutly, place the crystals on the paper. Now pick up your pen again; it is time to use the power of creativity to bring a protective symbol, or

sigil, to life. There is no wrong way to do this, so do not feel self-doubt. Rely on the energy of the crystals to guide you.

✦ Rearrange the consonants as you rewrite them, linking them to form a symbol. Perhaps you arrange them in a circular fashion to encourage holistic protection. Or maybe you draw them in a line or arrow shape to encourage pointed protection. Let your inner witch and the needs of your group be the guide.

✦ When you have created a sigil you are happy with (don't be afraid to go through a few drafts!), take a new sheet of paper and write the final version of the sigil on it. Seal the protective power of the sigil by brushing the sprig of parsley like a paintbrush over the lines of the newly created sigil.

✦ Use this sigil on group documents, materials, walls, or in your own Book of Shadows to afford constant protection to the group and to heal incoming negative energy.

JAR FULL OF HARMONY

PURPOSE OF SPELL: This jar potion will heal general discord in the group and encourage vibes of harmony.

SUGGESTED TIMING:
Waxing moon

ITEMS NEEDED:
• Glass jar with lid

MAGICKAL INGREDIENTS:
• 1 cup dried chamomile
• 1 teaspoon nutmeg
• 1 sodalite crystal
• 1 clear quartz crystal
• 6 drops tea tree oil

SPELLWORK

✦ Arrange the dried chamomile in a circular fashion, lining the inside bottom rim of the jar to form a complete circle, focusing your intention on calming balance and harmony.

✦ Sprinkle the nutmeg into the jar, focusing on connection and understanding.

✦ Place three drops of tea tree oil inside the jar, on the right side; do the same on the left side of the jar, focusing on balance and clearing of negative energy.

✦ Finish the charm by placing the sodalite and the clear quartz in the center of the jar. Cover the jar to seal the energy of the elements together. Leave the jar by a window to magickally charge through the night of the full moon.

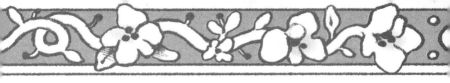

✦ Place the magickally charged jar on your altar, desk, or in a group communal area to emanate vibes of healing harmony. Take the cover off for an extra boost. Refresh each month as needed.

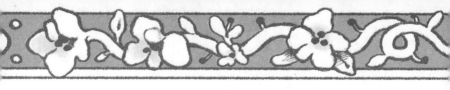

POWER OF THREE FOR ENERGY

PURPOSE OF SPELL: This spell invokes candle magick to heal low energy with an invigorating energy transfer. Use this spell to heal groups suffering from mental and physical fatigue.

SUGGESTED TIMING:
Waxing moon, full moon

ITEMS NEEDED:

- 3 candles
- 1 plate
- Lighter

MAGICKAL INGREDIENTS:

- ½ cup dried rosemary
- ½ cup dried mint
- Eucalyptus oil (as needed)

SPELLWORK

✦ Anoint each candle with a few drops of eucalyptus oil for a boost of invigorating energy.

✦ Mix the rosemary and mint and cover your plate with it evenly. Roll each oiled candle in the mix to dress the candle with strength and renewal.

✦ Stand your candles up on your altar and incant while lighting:

"As one candle shines so very bright,
Let rejuvenation flow and ignite.
As two candles shine together so strong,
Let energy rise and low vibration be gone.

THE HEALING POWER OF WITCHCRAFT

As three candles shine in harmony,
Let strength stay, so mote it be."

✦ Let the candles burn for at least 3 minutes as you meditate on the growing energy. When ready, blow them out. Store the candles upright in a cool, dry location and bring them out to light whenever your group needs an influx of energy. Refresh the oil and herbs as needed.

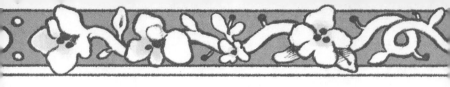

LEAD WITH LOVE CHARM

PURPOSE OF SPELL: This charm will help the group reach for the strength of love when interacting with each other. This charm will help heal ego weaknesses that send group members into conflict.

SUGGESTED TIMING:
Full moon

ITEMS NEEDED:
- String or ribbon for hanging
- Two 12-inch lengths of ribbon

MAGICKAL INGREDIENTS:
- 7 sprigs of fresh rosemary
- 1 small clear quartz crystal

SPELLWORK

✦ Lay out the sprigs of rosemary on your altar.

✦ Gather them into a bundle one at a time, incanting:

> *"Sprig of one for conflict undone*
> *Sprig of two to see it through*
> *Sprig of three to calm rough seas*
> *Sprig of four to let love soar*
> *Sprig of five and healing arrives*
> *Sprig of six all conflicts fix*
> *Sprig of seven the past forgiven."*

✦ Tie the sprigs together with the two ribbons wrapped securely around the base of the bundle to bind the spell.

✦ Nestle the small clear quartz crystal between the ribbon and the rosemary to amplify the power of the charm.

✦ Hang in a prominent location such as above a door or in a window as a reminder of the charm's power.

TWO SIDES BECOME ONE

PURPOSE OF SPELL: This spell is meant to bring opposing viewpoints together and heal the indifference and tension two sides hold for each other.

SUGGESTED TIMING:
New moon, waxing moon

ITEMS NEEDED:

- 2 small bowls filled with salt
- Candle
- Lighter
- Medium-sized bowl
- Jar with lid

MAGICKAL INGREDIENTS:

- 1 bay leaf
- 1 tablespoon ground turmeric
- 1 tablespoon ground cayenne pepper

SPELLWORK

✦ Place the two bowls of salt on either side of your candle. Each bowl represents one side in the conflict.

✦ Add the turmeric powder on top of the salt in the right-hand bowl, and add the cayenne on top of the salt in the left-hand bowl. Consider how similar the two spices appear even though they are very different.

✦ Place your finger in the center of the turmeric/salt and make a spiral leading outward in a clockwise motion. Do the same with the cayenne/salt mixture, but this time spiral your finger counterclockwise.

✦ Light your candle and incant:

"Now two sides, different in makeup but still so alike,
Will come together by the flame of this light."

✦ Combine the two small bowls into the medium-sized bowl. Using your finger, create a pentagram in the mixture to bind the two sides together.

✦ Light the bay leaf in the candle flame and let it burn over the bowl to seal your healing intention. As the lit bay leaf reaches your fingers, drop the remaining burning leaf into the salt mixture. Use the lighter to finish burning any remaining bay leaf.

✦ Place the mixture in a jar and securely close it with a lid. Store in a harmonious location like among house plants, near a warm fireplace, or by a pleasant window until the full moon. On the morning after the full moon, discard the jar's contents in an outside bin to complete the magickal healing of discord between two opposing sides.

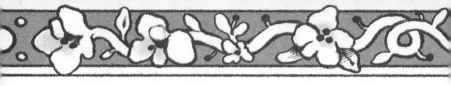

DISPERSE AND DEFEAT INJUSTICE

PURPOSE OF SPELL: This spell protects those faced with injustices and helps heal the groups affected.

SUGGESTED TIMING:
Full moon

ITEMS NEEDED:
- Cauldron
- Boiling water
- Piece of paper
- Pen with black ink

MAGICKAL INGREDIENTS:
- 2 tablespoons ground sage
- 1 black tourmaline crystal
- 1 clear quartz crystal

SPELLWORK

✦ Write down the injustices the group is facing on the piece of paper.

✦ Lay the list in the empty cauldron and weight it down with the strengthening, pain-absorbing tourmaline and the amplifying clear quartz. Sprinkle the sage over the paper with clearing intention.

✦ When ready, pour the boiling water into the cauldron, over the paper. Watch the ink disperse as the healing water hits it. Feel the crystals absorbing the negative energy released from the paper. Smell the sage, cleansing, soothing, and healing. As the water penetrates, so does healing energy. As the water cools, so does the power of injustice.

✦ When the water is fully cooled, retrieve your crystals from the cauldron for cleansing. Discard the remaining contents of the cauldron into the toilet to send injustice far away from the group, where it belongs.

FIVE SENSES OF TOLERANCE

PURPOSE OF SPELL: Oftentimes groups consist of many different types of people, some who have life experiences and backgrounds completely different from our own. This ritual heals any lingering intolerance we may harbor and attunes our bodies to compassion for otherness.

SUGGESTED TIMING:
As needed

ITEMS NEEDED:

- Small bowl
- Cotton swab
- ½ ounce jojoba oil

MAGICKAL INGREDIENTS:

- 7 drops tea tree oil or lavender oil, whichever scent you prefer

SPELLWORK

✦ Mix your oils thoroughly in a small bowl with a cotton swab. Replenish the amount of oil if needed throughout this ritual.

✦ Incant:

> *"I am but one person, a part of the whole*
> *Tolerance and compassion is my goal."*

✦ Carefully dab the oil between your eyes and on your forehead and say:

> *"Open my eyes so I may see value in otherness.*
> *By this oil I banish indifference."*

✦ Carefully dab the oil on each earlobe and say:

> *"Open my ears so I may hear the truth of others.*
> *By this oil we support one another."*

✦ Carefully dab oil on your upper lip area between your nose and mouth. Use very sparingly if you are sensitive to smells. Say:

> *"Open my nose so I may sniff out intolerance.*
> *By this oil I welcome aberrance."*

✦ Carefully dab the oil on your chin and say:

> *"Open my mouth to speak compassion to difference.*
> *By this oil my kindness is vociferous."*

✦ Carefully dab the oil on each wrist and say:

> *"Open my touch to be caring and kind.*
> *By this oil tolerance I bind."*

✦ Allow the calming scent to break down any energy barriers and rejuvenate your commitment to tolerance.

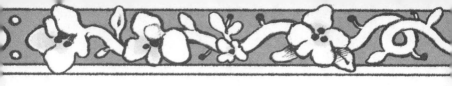

HELPING HAND WASH

PURPOSE OF SPELL: This spell encourages the group to help and support each other and heals "lone wolf" attitudes that can hinder productivity and creativity.

SUGGESTED TIMING:
As needed

ITEMS NEEDED:

- Large bowl big enough to comfortably fit both hands in
- Warm water

MAGICKAL INGREDIENTS:

- ½ cup fresh basil leaves
- Green aventurine crystals
- Smoky quartz crystals
- A few drops orange oil

SPELLWORK

✦ Place the crystals in the center of your bowl.

✦ Pour the water over the crystals and let the water charge for a minute. Add the basil and orange to the bowl of water with the intention of joyous, supportive relationships.

✦ Immerse both your hands in the water. Make washing motions with your hands to clear away unhelpful energy. Comb the water with your fingers and tell it how calming it is. Cup the water and let it drop while telling the water how supportive it is. Splash a bit. Be playful and friendly with the water. This water is all about connection and positivity. Meditate on your group members and think of ways you can be of service to each other.

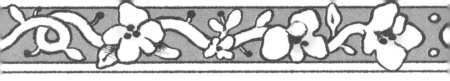

✦ Enjoy the water until it cools. Remove your hands and discard the water. Continue your work with refreshed, helping hands and know through sympathy magick the handwash is helping your group as well.

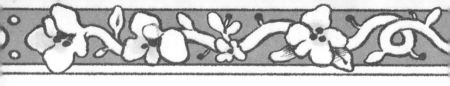

LEADING THE WAY

PURPOSE OF SPELL: This spell strengthens group leaders, healing self-doubt and assuaging ego with an understanding heart. Use candle magick to help light a righteous path for group leadership.

SUGGESTED TIMING:
Full moon

ITEMS NEEDED:

- 3 candles
- Lighter
- Cauldron

MAGICKAL INGREDIENTS:

- Sprig of dried thyme
- Sprig of dried lavender
- Sprig of dried rosemary
- 1 green aventurine crystal
- 1 amethyst crystal
- 1 citrine crystal

SPELLWORK

✦ Place the three candles on your altar, side by side.

✦ Place the aventurine in front of one candle to represent a compassionate heart.

✦ Place the amethyst in front of the second candle to represent enduring wisdom.

✦ Place the citrine in front of the third candle to represent mindful action.

✦ Light all three candles and say:

> *"By power of three and three again,*
> *I send healing to leadership. Now it begins."*

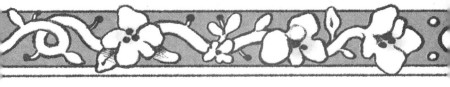

✦ Burn the thyme on the first candle and say:

"Leaves of thyme, burn today, any ego that stands in the way."

Drop the burning thyme in your cauldron as it reaches **your** fingers.

✦ Burn the lavender sprig on the second candle and say:

"Lavender stalk burning bright, give wisdom's spark eternal light."

Drop the burning lavender in your cauldron as it reaches your fingers.

✦ Burn the rosemary sprig on the third candle and say:

"Rosemary branch lit with flame, let mindful action lead the day."

Drop the burning rosemary in your cauldron as it reaches your fingers.

✦ Once the herbal contents of the cauldron stop burning, **blow** out your candles to seal the spell. Scatter ashes outside, **binding** the magick to earth for strength.

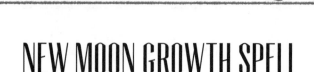

NEW MOON GROWTH SPELL

PURPOSE OF SPELL: Sometimes we just can't seem to make headway or grow in our work. This spell uses new moon magick to cast off the previous moon cycle's disappointments. It also heals any resulting bitterness so groups may move forward in a robust, growth mindset.

SUGGESTED TIMING:
New moon

ITEMS NEEDED:

- 4 candles
- Lighter
- Athame

MAGICKAL INGREDIENTS:

- Amethyst crystals
- Fluorite crystals

SPELLWORK

✦ Carve the symbols for the elements into the candles. Use one element symbol on each candle.

✦ Place the earth candle to the north on your altar, the air candle to the east, the fire candle to the south, and the water candle to the west.

✦ Place amethyst and fluorite in the crossroads center of the four candles.

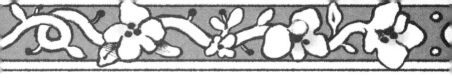

✦ Light the four candles and incant:

> *"By north, east, south, and west,*
> *I light this dark and moonless night.*
> *By east, south, west, and north, new energy shall be brought forth.*
> *By south, west, north, and east, last moon cycle is now released.*
> *By west, north, east, and south,*
> *Positive growth is now announced."*

✦ Meditate on all old energy clearing. Allow new growth-oriented energy to fill the space left by the banished failure and bitterness.

ALL WORK AND NO PLAY REMEDY

PURPOSE OF SPELL: Often groups work so hard toward goals, the group forgets to celebrate achievements. Use this spell to heal day-to-day drudgery and encourage a burst of creativity and fun.

SUGGESTED TIMING:
Full moon

ITEMS NEEDED:

- Your favorite booty-shaking playlist
- Essential oil diffuser
- Bubbles
- Candles

MAGICKAL INGREDIENTS:

- Carnelian crystals
- Rose quartz crystals
- Tourmaline crystals
- Essential oil blend:
  8 drops ylang-ylang oil,
  6 drop bergamot oil,
  4 drops orange oil

SPELLWORK

✦ Turn on your music and your essential oil diffuser with the blend in it.

✦ Set up candles and crystals all over your chosen space. You want to fill the night with light and pretty things to lift your mood. Dance it out as you set up a beautiful area to enjoy.

✦ When ready, take out the bubbles. Blow one bubble for each member of your group. As you watch the bubbles swirl, call out their name in joy. Continue to dance and enjoy the energy of your space for as long as it takes to feel your doldrums chased away by joy and creativity. Your new attitude will be infectious to your group the next time you see them.

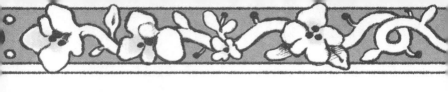

MAGICK WATER FOR A COMMUNITY GARDEN

PURPOSE OF SPELL: This spell heals any energy interference with the growth of a healthy community garden and promotes cooperation among the members.

SUGGESTED TIMING:
Waxing moon, full moon

MAGICKAL INGREDIENTS:

- ½ cup rosemary
- ½ cup basil
- Aventurine crystals
- Rose quartz crystals

ITEMS NEEDED:

- Large jar with lid
- Fresh water from multiple sources

SPELLWORK

✦ During the period of the waxing moon, make it your mission to collect water from three different sources in your community. Perhaps you use a friendly neighbor's garden hose or sink. Maybe there is a lake in your area or you find a running creek or river nearby. Another way to collect local water is setting out a bowl to collect rainwater in various locations.

✦ Mix all types of water in the large jar as you collect them.

✦ When all water is collected, add in the crystals and herbs.

✦ Set the water out to charge every night through the full moon. Swirl the contents to keep them flowing and activated daily. Once the full moon has passed, bring the water to your community garden and water your communal plants with it to promote growth, healing, and community service.

✦ Leave the crystals in the garden near any plants that could use an extra healing boost.

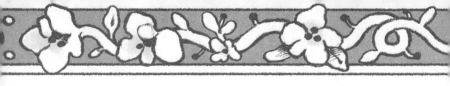

LEAVES OF TREES FOR COMMUNITY

PURPOSE OF SPELL: Our neighborhood communities are as diverse as the tree population. Use the power of healing trees to create a potion to bind the local community together and disperse feelings of isolation and loneliness.

SUGGESTED TIMING:
Waning moon, new moon

ITEMS NEEDED:

- Large baking tray
- Glass jar with lid
- Local tree leaves
- Mortar and pestle

MAGICKAL INGREDIENTS:

- Clear quartz crystals
- Rose quartz crystals
- Jasper crystals

SPELLWORK

✦ Collect 1 to 2 cups of varying types of leaves, foraged from your local outdoors. Spread them on a large tray so they are not layered. Place clear quartz and rose quartz crystals on top or among the leaves to charge them with loving, communal healing energy as they dry. Let them dry in a sunny, indoor location for a week or so.

✦ Once the leaves are dried, use your pestle to crush them all together in your mortar until they are just small flakes.

✦ As you grind, incant:

> *"Trees of plenty, leaves of love,*
> *Send us blessings from above.*
> *Strengthen this neighborhood and community*
> *Connect us all with loving and healing energy."*

✦ Pour the ground leaves into your jar. Top the leaves with jasper crystals to anchor the potion to the community. **Bring the jar with you on a walk around your neighborhood so the** healing magick may emanate far and wide.

THE MAGICK CHAIN OF SERVICE

PURPOSE OF SPELL: This charm will create cohesion between the group and the community it serves, healing any blockages in working together for the common good.

SUGGESTED TIMING:
Full moon

ITEMS NEEDED:
- Small bowl
- Four 8.5-by-11-inch pieces of construction paper
- Scissors

ITEMS CONT.
- Coloring markers
- Tape
- Cotton swab
- ½ ounce jojoba oil

MAGICKAL INGREDIENTS:
- 4 drops cedar oil

SPELLWORK

✦ Mix the cedar and jojoba oil in a small bowl using a cotton swab. Charge the mixture by drawing a pentagram in it with the swab.

✦ Cut each piece of paper into four strips lengthwise. The strips should measure about 2 by 11 inches.

✦ You now have 16 pieces of paper. Four is a number of structural cohesion, and we will use the power of this number squared to build a 16-piece magickal chain. On each strip of paper, write a different project, campaign, facet, program, or tool of the organization and how it is meant to aid the community.

✦ When finished writing, dip your cotton swab in the oil mixture. Dab the oiled cotton swab lightly over each of the 16 messages to seal the intention.

✦ Create a paper chain with the strips of paper. As you build the chain, chant:

"Four by four, we build foundation
Four by four, we add connection
Four by four, we help and aid
Four by four, community made."

✦ Hang the chain on display to radiate healing community service energy.

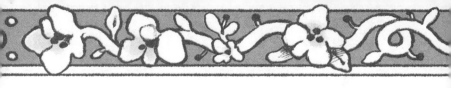

GROUP SPELL FOR HEALING, GROWTH, AND WHOLENESS

PURPOSE OF SPELL: This is a group spell you may perform with friends, family, a coven, or an organization to connect the group in healing prayer.

SUGGESTED TIMING:
Full moon

ITEMS NEEDED:
- Essential oil diffuser
- 1 candle for each participant
- Lighter

ITEMS CONT.
- Prayer card with written incantation for those who are not familiar with the prayer

MAGICKAL INGREDIENTS:
- Essential oil blend:
  8 drops ylang-ylang oil,
  8 drops bergamot oil

SPELLWORK

✦ Turn on the diffuser with the oil blend.

✦ Form a circle with each participant sitting cross-legged on the ground. Give each participant a candle that they may lay on the floor in front of their feet, pointing inward. Participants should sit close together and place their hands on the knee of the person to the left and right of them. Right arm is the over arm, left arm is the under arm.

✦ The leader leads a short breathing exercise to synchronize the energy in the room and says:

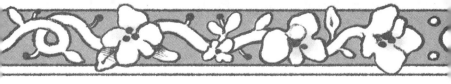

"Breathe in healing, hold, breathe out pain.
Breathe in love, hold, breathe out hate.
Breathe in the positive, hold, breathe out the negative.
Breathe in self-confidence, hold, breathe out doubt."

✦ The leader releases their hands from their neighbors' knees and signals everyone else may do the same. The leader then picks up their candle and lights it. The leader turns to the person on their left and lights their candle from the flame of the first candle. This person then lights the candle of the person to the left of them with their own newly lit candle. Continue lighting, candle to candle, around the circle until all candles are lit.

LEADER: *"We ask for healing energy."*

GROUP: *"Cleanse us. Cure us. Restore us."*

LEADER: *"We ask for strength and growth."*

GROUP: *"Steady us. Fortify us. Nourish us."*

LEADER: *"We ask for compassion and an open heart."*

GROUP: *"Love us. Ground us. Grow us."*

ALL: Blow out candles.

LEADER: *"We go forth to live the energy we have created here together."*

GROUP: *"So mote it be."*

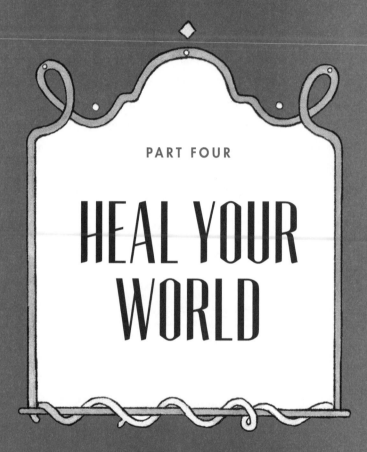

PART FOUR

HEAL YOUR WORLD

WITCHES DRAW ENERGY FROM THEIR SUR-roundings and are affected greatly by the energies we immerse ourselves in. We have homes we seek shelter in. We have a planet we steward. We care for these places as an act of care for ourselves and others we live alongside. The empathetic, sympathetic nature of witch-craft is best served by spaces that support clear, posi-tive, growth-oriented, healing energies. By healing the energies in our homes, outdoor spaces, and the planet as a whole, our power base strengthens and deepens exponentially through our families, communities, and humankind. Here are spells and rituals that show you how to heal your home and the planet and achieve lasting healing energy for the greatest good—that is, a world full of healed healers who change the course of energy to heal our Mother Earth forever.

HEAL YOUR HOME

A witch's home is our sanctuary and our power base. We draw energy from the environments we create for ourselves, and that energy should match our healing intentions. The spells and rituals that follow heal your home of negative influences and protect your home from possible negative infiltrates. The goal of these magickal workings is to conjure a peaceful, healing environment you may rely on to support your magickal healing endeavors.

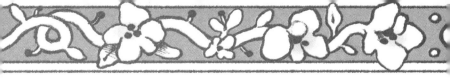

WELCOMING LAVENDER DOOR WASH

PURPOSE OF SPELL: This spell heals your home of any unwelcoming vibes and promotes an aura of joyful salutation to visitors.

SUGGESTED TIMING:
New moon

ITEMS NEEDED:

- Large bowl of hot water
- Washcloth

MAGICKAL INGREDIENTS:

- 5 sprigs of fresh lavender or 1 cup dried lavender
- 3 drops lavender essential oil

SPELLWORK

✦ A witch's door is traditionally painted purple. Harness the power of your witchy entranceway by washing it in purple lavender, the herb of warmth and welcome.

✦ Add all your ingredients to the hot water.

✦ Allow them to magickally infuse the water as you incant:

> *"Lavender purple, warm and true.*
> *Create welcoming vibes anew."*

CONTINUED >>>

✦ Dip your washcloth in the water and wipe down your entire front door with the welcoming, witchy water. Know you are chasing away any unwelcoming vibes and healing your door as a portal to sanctuary. When finished, pour any remaining water and herbs onto your front stoop or hide the herbs under your welcome mat for a lasting sense of welcoming energy.

WITCH DOOR BELLS

PURPOSE OF SPELL: Create a witchy bell charm to hang on the doorknob of your home. The bells will ring each time someone enters or exits, and their energy will be cleansed as they do so. This will heal your home of incoming negative energy and release your guest's energy from your home as they leave.

SUGGESTED TIMING:
Full moon

ITEMS NEEDED:
- 3 decorative ribbons
- 3 bells

MAGICKAL INGREDIENTS:
- Orange oil
- Frankincense oil
- Cedar oil

SPELLWORK

✦ Lay out the three ribbons on your altar. One represents friendship and goodwill. The second represents cleansing and purification. The third represents grounding and calm. Tie them all together by one end, leaving the other ends free. Dab one drop of each oil on the knot.

✦ Next, attach one bell to the free end of each ribbon. Take the friendship ribbon and dab sweet orange oil on the bell knot. Take the cleansing ribbon and dab frankincense oil on the bell knot. On the final grounding ribbon, dab cedar oil on the bell knot.

CONTINUED >>>

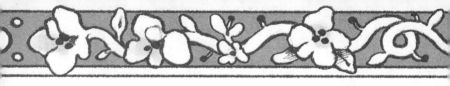

✦ Loop the ribbon tops around the indoor knob to your front door and knot them tightly to the knob stem. Your doorway will now be consistently healed of negative energy and will promote friendship, good cheer, and solid grounding for all who enter your home.

CLEARWATER HEARTH MAGICK

PURPOSE OF SPELL: This spell uses hearth magick of a stovetop boil to purify your home's air and heal lingering negative energies. The resulting potion is strained of all materials to give the appearance of regular water again, but it is actually a secret, protective wash. Hence the name, Clearwater.

SUGGESTED TIMING:
Waning moon, new moon

ITEMS NEEDED:

- Stovetop
- Medium-sized saucepan with lid
- 3 cups water
- Large spoon for stirring
- Pasta strainer
- Large jar or empty plastic milk jug rinsed well

ITEMS CONT.

- Cloth or rag
- Pinch of salt
- 1 whole lemon

MAGICKAL INGREDIENTS:

- 1 cup fresh sage leaf
- 3 sprigs of fresh rosemary
- 1 tablespoon grated ginger

SPELLWORK

✦ Cut your lemon widthwise into eight slivers to draw power from the eight phases of the moon.

✦ Pour the three cups of water into your saucepan. Add the sage, rosemary, lemon, ginger, and a pinch of salt to the water.

CONTINUED >>>

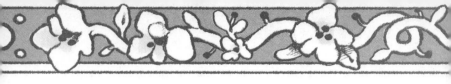

✦ Allow the ingredients to come to a boil together on medium-high heat. Stir the potion occasionally with your spoon as it heats.

✦ Once the water is rapidly boiling, turn down the heat to low and partially cover the pot with the lid.

✦ Let the pot simmer for a few hours, gently turning up the heat again if more energy is needed. You may also remove the cover for a more robust-smelling potion. The scent will purify your home through air magick of steam.

✦ When done simmering, let the mixture cool. Strain the mixture into the empty bottle. Compost or discard the herbs and fruit. Store the Clearwater away from sunlight.

✦ Use the water on a rag to wipe down windows, door thresholds, or individual objects like crystals that require purification and protection. You may also use this water on yourself by dabbing it on your forehead daily for protection or adding it to a purification bath. Clearwater clears negative energies and raises the level of protection, all while looking like a harmless jar of plain water.

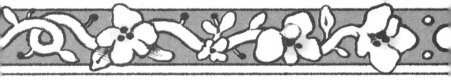

THREE NIGHTS TO A DECLUTTERED HOME

PURPOSE OF SPELL: This spell will help heal the home of clutter that often signals ego attachment and blocks productive spellwork with its overwhelming energy.

SUGGESTED TIMING:
New moon

ITEMS NEEDED:
- Essential oil diffuser
- Two large boxes
- Marker
- Candle
- Lighter

MAGICKAL INGREDIENTS:
- Citrine crystals
- Black tourmaline crystals
- Essential oil blend:
  5 drops eucalyptus oil,
  5 drops peppermint oil,
  5 drops orange oil

SPELLWORK

✦ The new moon period lasts three nights. To not overwhelm yourself, select three areas of the home to declutter during this period. Perhaps you'll choose a bookshelf, your clothes closet, and your whole kitchen. Focus on spaces that will make a meaningful difference in your day-to-day sense of calm and focus.

CONTINUED >>>

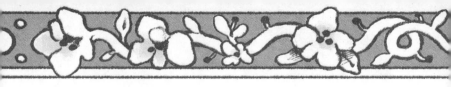

✦ Start on the first night of the new moon. Turn on your essential oil diffuser with the blend in the area you are working. Light a candle close by, but not in your way of working. Surround the candle with citrine and tourmaline crystals. Between the energy of the clearing new moon, the oil blend, and the candle/crystals mini-altar, you are well armed with productive energy to let things go.

✦ Bring out your two large boxes. On one box draw a large spiral counterclockwise. This box will be for things you are going to throw away, recycle, compost, or donate. On the other box draw a spiral clockwise. This box will be for things you want to keep and need to find storage for.

✦ Turn on some uplifting music and give it your best effort for an hour. Repeat each night of the new moon. You will be in awe of how much you can get done in three hours to reveal a newly refreshed space. Enjoy the freedom and energy the decluttered spaces will bring you and your magickal workings.

PROTECTIVE PENTAGRAM CHARM

PURPOSE OF SPELL: This spell uses the five sides of the pentagram to shine protective energy into all areas of your home and heal those spaces of negative energies as needed.

SUGGESTED TIMING:
Full moon

ITEMS NEEDED:

- 5 sticks of equal length and width, foraged from outside
- Twine or ribbon
- Scissors

MAGICKAL INGREDIENTS:

- 1 green aventurine crystal
- 1 jasper crystal
- 1 carnelian crystal
- 1 sodalite crystal
- 1 amethyst crystal
- Cedar oil (as needed)
- Frankincense oil (as needed)

SPELLWORK

✦ On the night of the full moon, anoint each of your sticks with a small amount of cedar and frankincense oil.

✦ Place one stick in the garden, on the porch, on the front stoop, or in another secure outdoor area of your home alongside the green aventurine crystal.

✦ Place the second stick on a main kitchen counter alongside the jasper.

CONTINUED >>>

✦ Place the third stick on your fireplace mantel or in your living room alongside the carnelian.

✦ Place the fourth stick in the bathroom you use most often alongside the sodalite.

✦ Place the fifth stick under your bed alongside the amethyst.

✦ Let all sticks rest in their location overnight, soaking in the full moon energy, the energy of the room they are presiding over, and the energy of the crystals and oils.

✦ In the morning, bind all the sticks together in the shape of a pentagram with twine or ribbon. This will seal all parts of your home's energy together. Hang the newly created pentagram of protection and healing over the front door of your house.

WITCHY WORKSPACE MAKEOVER

PURPOSE OF SPELL: Adorn your desk or workspace with the healing magick of thyme, crystals, and aromatherapy to draw strength and concentration to your work.

SUGGESTED TIMING:
New moon

ITEMS NEEDED:
- Essential oil diffuser
- Sunny window

MAGICKAL INGREDIENTS:
- Potted thyme plant
- Citrine crystals
- Green aventurine crystals
- Carnelian crystals
- Essential oil blend:
  8 drops peppermint oil,
  8 drops frankincense oil

SPELLWORK

✦ Place the thyme plant in a sunny location where it may flourish and where you can work.

✦ Fill the diffuser with the essential oil blend and turn it on for 15-minute intervals while you work.

✦ Intersperse your workspace with citrine for willpower, aventurine for work that flows from the heart, and carnelian for creativity and passion.

✦ Hold the crystals, turn on your diffuser, and enjoy the strength of your thyme plant when you are feeling low on energy, focus, or concentration.

SALTY HEARTH WITCHERY

PURPOSE OF SPELL: These salt bowl charms are the perfect way to be proactive about potential negative energy by setting them out in your hearth and living spaces to collect negative energy as it arises. They are healing helpers, waiting in the wings.

SUGGESTED TIMING:
Create each new moon, discard monthly and refresh

ITEMS NEEDED:

* Multiple small bowls or glassware, as many as there are rooms in your home
* At least 1 pound salt

MAGICKAL INGREDIENTS:

* Whole cloves
* Clear quartz crystals
* Black tourmaline crystals
* Fluorite crystals
* Tea tree oil or frankincense oil for each bowl or cup, whichever scent you prefer

SPELLWORK

✦ Line your bowls or cups with salt, at least 1 inch deep.

✦ Add an energy-absorbing crystal like clear quartz, tourmaline, or fluorite to the center.

✦ Add a small amount of clove on top of the salt.

✦ Add a few drops of oil to seal the mixture.

✦ Place your creations in discreet but high-trafficked areas of your house, in every room if possible, to proactively heal incoming negative energy.

REFLECTIONS ON COMFORT

PURPOSE OF SPELL: This spell will emanate vibes of comfort throughout your home on days when you are feeling on edge or not well. Let the healing powers of light and aroma calm and comfort your space to soothe your spirit.

SUGGESTED TIMING:
As needed

ITEMS NEEDED:

- Small bowl
- Cotton swab
- ½ ounce jojoba oil
- 1 large mirror
- 5 candles

ITEMS CONT.

- Cauldron lined with salt
- Lighter
- 1 large tray (a large cutting board, cheese board, or baking pan works well)

MAGICKAL INGREDIENTS:

- 5 dried bay leaves
- 5 drops lavender essential oil

SPELLWORK

✦ Mix the jojoba oil and lavender oil together in the small bowl with the cotton swab. Use the oiled swab to draw a large pentagram on the tray with the lavender oil mixture. Let each line of the pentagram represent an area of discomfort you are targeting to assuage with this spell. Place the tray in front of a large mirror.

CONTINUED >>>

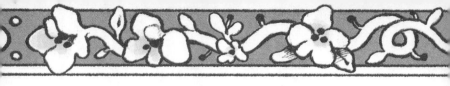

✦ Stand your candles in front of the mirror on the tray. Each candle should cover one tip of the oil five-pointed star.

✦ Light your candles and incant:

"By one candle and then two,
I call this spell to reflect clear and true.
By candle three and then four,
I encourage comfort from ceiling to floor.
This last candle lit of five,
Soothes my spirits and cleanses the vibe."

✦ One by one, burn the bay leaves on the flames. Be sure to drop the bay leaf in the cauldron as it reaches your fingers or use tongs to avoid the flame. As you burn each bay leaf, speak aloud the intentioned area of discomfort in your life you are releasing. Focus your intention on letting go of agitation. Breathe deeply the comforting aroma of burning bay leaf.

✦ Once you are done burning all bay leaves, focus on the candles glowing in your mirror. Allow their calming light to wash over you and fill the spaces you just released with healing, comforting energy.

THE HEALING POWER OF WITCHCRAFT

GARLAND OF JOY

PURPOSE OF SPELL: This charm, popular at Yuletide for bringing good cheer, is a wonderful way to bring the energy of joy and camaraderie into your home all year long. Help heal sorrow, depression, and worry by creating a happiness garland to hang in your kitchen window.

SUGGESTED TIMING:
Waxing moon, full moon

ITEMS NEEDED:

- 1 to 2 oranges, depending on their size
- Length of twine, about 6 to 12 inches longer than the width of your kitchen window
- Additional ribbon to attach dangling rosemary and cinnamon

ITEMS CONT.

- Toothpick or kebab skewer
- Cookie drying racks
- Thumbtacks

MAGICKAL INGREDIENTS:

- ½ cup whole star anise
- 3 sprigs of rosemary
- 3 cinnamon sticks

SPELLWORK

DRY THE ORANGE SLICES

✦ Before you are able to string the garland, you must first dry your oranges. The heat of the oven will secure the magickal joy–filled properties of the fruit for much longer than a fresh orange.

✦ Preheat your oven to 250°F.

CONTINUED >>>

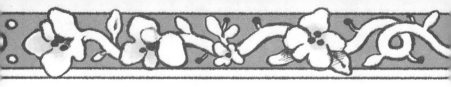

✦ Slice your orange into ½- to ¼-inch-thick pieces. Pierce a hole in the center of each orange slice with a toothpick or skewer. Lay the slices on cookie drying racks (not a baking pan) to prevent stickage. Bake at 250°F for 2 to 3 hours, turning every 30 minutes or so to ensure evenness. If you have a convection oven, they may be done more quickly, so keep an eye on them as they begin to brown. Remove from the oven when ready and let them cool completely.

CRAFT YOUR GARLAND

✦ Time to get creative! Gather your materials to craft the garland. Feel free to add your own ingredients like pine cones or crystals if you so desire.

✦ String the twine with alternating materials as pleases you. Start with a dried orange slice. Next, add one or a few whole star anises. Add all orange slices and star anise, alternating as you go. Drape the garland from one end of your kitchen window to the other, securing with thumbtacks to the wall.

✦ Finish your creation by tying sprigs of rosemary and cinnamon sticks as dangling charms off the garland twine.

✦ Enjoy the amazing scents and joyful energy as sadness is lifted and worries healed. Discard after a few weeks and create again if you so desire.

BLACK SALT FOR BAD VIBES

PURPOSE OF SPELL: This spell creates black salt, which is a ritual salt used to heal negative energy and protect the home from negative entities.

SUGGESTED TIMING:
Full moon

ITEMS NEEDED:
- ½ cup salt (preferably white sea salt)
- Mortar and pestle
- Jar

MAGICKAL INGREDIENTS:
- 1 tablespoon pepper
- 2 tablespoons ash from your magickal workings

SPELLWORK

✦ You may secure the ash from the remains of a fire in your fireplace, a bonfire, or after you burn ritual herbs. Avoid ash with wax from candle drippings in it to keep the mixture pure.

✦ Combine ingredients in your mortar and grind them with the pestle until everything is well mixed, at least 5 minutes.

CONTINUED >>>

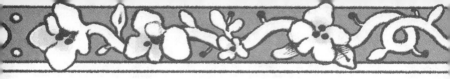

✦ As you grind, incant:

> *"Turn now, salt, I command to thee*
> *By pepper, by ash, thy property*
> *Become a powerful shield, steadfast and strong*
> *Your bid is now mine, black salt be born."*

✦ Store the ritual salt in the jar. Sprinkle a bit of black salt every full moon on the entranceways of your home. You may also sprinkle some on the floor after a bad fight or illness occurs in the house to absorb negative energy. Simply vacuum it up after 30 minutes or so and discard the vacuum contents in an outdoor bin.

HEALING GARDEN PENTAGRAM

PURPOSE OF SPELL: Harness the healing power of five powerful garden plants by creating a pentagram of healing elemental energy in your garden.

SUGGESTED TIMING:
Plant in the spring during a new moon after the danger of frost has passed.

ITEMS NEEDED:
- Gardening trowel
- Garden pavers (optional)

MAGICKAL INGREDIENTS:
- Thyme plant
- Rosemary plant
- Basil plant
- Sage plant
- Oregano plant
- 5 green aventurine crystals

SPELLWORK

✦ Create a magickal pentagram oasis in your garden by strategically planting these five plants. I recommend using plants at least 6 to 8 inches high.

✦ Begin by plotting out a pentagram in your garden by drawing the lines with your gardening trowel. Dig holes for the plants at the tip of each star point. You want the plants to be about 2 to 3 feet apart.

✦ Plant the thyme plant in the top point of the star to symbolize your witchy spirit that needs strength and healing from time to time.

CONTINUED >>>

✦ Plant the rosemary on the point of the star in the three o'clock position. Rosemary is known as "the dew of the sea" and invokes healing water vibes.

✦ Plant the basil, an herb with fire correspondence, in the five o'clock position to invoke the healing properties of fire.

✦ Plant the sage, an herb with earthy correspondence, in the seven o'clock position to invoke the healing properties of earth.

✦ Plant the oregano, an herb with air correspondence, in the nine o'clock position to invoke the healing properties of air.

✦ Bless and encourage each newly planted herb by placing stones of green aventurine at their base.

✦ Add garden pavers to delineate the sides of the star if you desire a more pronounced pentagram effect.

✦ Meditate often in the middle of your healing pentagram of plant energy to refresh, renew, and heal.

SANCTUARY OF PEACE

PURPOSE OF SPELL: It is not always possible to keep an entirely peaceful and healing vibe in your home, especially if we live with other people. From small children, to hormonal teenagers, to barking pets, to family members who may be having a bad day, your witchy self needs a source of healing escape. Use this ritual to create a sanctuary you may visit when your home's energy is chaotic.

SUGGESTED TIMING:
As needed

ITEMS NEEDED:
• Essential oil diffuser

MAGICKAL INGREDIENTS:
• 5 rosemary or lavender sprigs
• 1 rose quartz crystal
• 1 fluorite crystal
• 1 amethyst crystal
• Lavender essential oil

SPELLWORK

✦ Identify a small, out-of-the-way space for your sanctuary. Perhaps your bedroom or bathroom makes sense for you. Others may find comfort in areas by bookshelves or on an outdoor patio. I have even used a large linen closet for this purpose. Find a location that is right for you.

✦ Add a few drops of lavender oil to your diffuser and turn it on.

CONTINUED >>>

✦ Arrange your three crystals in front of you in the space you've chosen for yourself. Invoke the wisdom of the maiden, mother, and crone to help calm you if you so desire. Ask the rose quartz for the optimism of the maiden, the fluorite for the absorbent healing of the mother, and the amethyst for the wisdom of the crone.

✦ Breathe deeply and slowly as you meditate on drawing calm and peace to yourself. Give yourself the gift of letting go of every current worry and loud voice in your head. Just for now.

✦ Use your five herbal sprigs to lay a pentagram before yourself. As you place each sprig, feel yourself more connected to peace. Feel the peace grow as you complete the pentagram. Admire your creation with more deep breaths of the lavender oil. When ready, bring this energy back to the work and relationships of your day.

WITCH'S LADDER CHARM

PURPOSE OF SPELL: This charm helps emanate specific positive energies of your own choosing throughout your home. Oftentimes we feel overwhelmed by a lack of path or clarity in our lives. Building a witch's ladder to hang in your home helps heal this sense of directionlessness and builds the energy of the life you want to live among, absorb, and practice.

SUGGESTED TIMING:
Full moon

ITEMS NEEDED:

- 3 feet of ribbon or twine for your ladder rails
- Additional small bits of ribbon or twine to attach dangling charm rungs

MAGICKAL INGREDIENTS:

- Sprig of rosemary
- Clear quartz crystals
- 10 more small elements of your choosing

SPELLWORK

✦ This spell garners its power from your intentionality for your own life and from your knot magick. As such, you will begin the spell by choosing 10 elements you have on hand that reflect the type of energy you wish to draw to your home and your life. There is no wrong way to choose items. You simply want items that inspire and motivate you, and are small enough to be tied to your witch's ladder ribbon. Some examples of objects include:

CONTINUED >>>

- Seashells to harness the depths of oceanic, feminine wisdom.

- A mint sprig, coin, or dollar to draw money to your life.

- A rock from your garden to encourage groundedness.

- A crystal that resonates with what you are searching for, such as rose quartz for love or citrine for confidence.

- A feather to inspire your voice and opinions to be spoken and heard.

- A bell to clear stagnation.

- A pen, paintbrush, crochet needle, and so on, to encourage your artistic streak.

- A playing card or tarot card such as the Queen of Hearts/Cups that speaks to love.

- A necklace or charm from a loved one to heal bumps in your relationship.

✦ The possibilities are endless! What matters most is that the objects matter to you.

CREATE YOUR LADDER

✦ Lay out the 3 feet of twine horizontally across your workspace. This is your witch's ladder base, or rail.

✦ Begin by tying the sprig of rosemary and the clear quartz (flat pieces work best) to the center of your witch's ladder rail. This is your ladder's witchy power base. Continue by tying the remaining 10 objects on either side of the base, 5 on each side, dangling down from the rail. Spread them out as feels intuitively right to you.

✦ Once created, drape the ladder across a sunny window or hang straight down for a more discreet look. Either way, know these objects are working to heal specific obstacles you are facing in your life and sending you positive energy throughout your home to help you live with confidence to move forward.

INFUSE COOKING WITH HEALING LOVE

PURPOSE OF SPELL: As busy witches, we often find ourselves cooking meals in a hurry, not always having the time to place intentional magickal infusions of love and healing into our food. Create and hang this charm in your kitchen to steadily emanate healing vibes into your cooking and always keep mealtime infused with love.

SUGGESTED TIMING:
Full moon

ITEMS NEEDED:

- Muslin bag or cloth square
- Twine or ribbon

MAGICKAL INGREDIENTS:

- 3 fresh basil leaves
- 3 sprigs of mint
- 1 bay leaf
- 1 tablespoon allspice
- Rose quartz crystals
- Cedar oil (as needed)

SPELLWORK

✦ Add the herbs and spices to your bag. Top with rose quartz.

✦ Tie your bag closed with three knots. As you do, incant:

"Charm of love-filled energy, aid all cooking done by me.
In busy times and chaotic days,
Make meals of love today and always."

✦ Seal the charms by asperging a few drops of oil onto the knots. Charge the charm under the full moon. Hang in your kitchen near your cookspace to provide a constant flow of nourishing, healing love to your cooking. Refresh each full moon or as needed.

HOPES AND DREAMS RENEWED

PURPOSE OF SPELL: This spell, which may be performed as a group, is intended to release pessimism of your family unit that can disrupt the home's energy flow. By using the energizing fire and wish-granting bay leaf, your hopes and dreams are renewed.

SUGGESTED TIMING:
New moon

ITEMS NEEDED:

- Cauldron lined with 1 inch of salt
- Long lighter

MAGICKAL INGREDIENTS:

- 1 bay leaf for every major hope or dream you and your family hold

SPELLWORK

✦ Place the bowl of salt in the center of your family table. Gather around the table from all sides.

✦ Have each member stick their bay leaf in the salt so the leaf stands tall. One end should be anchored in the salt, and the other should stand straight up. As each member places their bay leaf, they should state their intention. For example, one may say, "I hope to hear positive news about my college admissions," or "I wish for peace from my anxiety." The group then repeats the

CONTINUED >>>

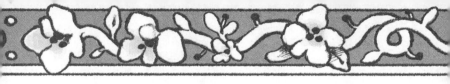

intention back to them with a unanimous voice of support. For example, "Fiona wishes to hear positive news about her college admissions."

✦ Once all leaves are placed with intention, each person, in turn, should use the long lighter to burn the leaves. Be sure to hold the lighter on the leaf until it is completely burned down to the salt. By the time you are done, the house should be pretty smoky, so be sure to open a window but also be sure to inhale the magickal goodness. This smoke will signal a healing release of your troubles and restore a sense of hope and faith in your dreams and goals.

HEAL THE PLANET

Due to a witch's reverence and connection to nature, it is essential to focus healing energy on our Mother Earth. We are stewards of the world's ecosystems, protectors of animals and plant life, and responders to Earth's natural disasters. As Thomas Moore wrote, "Earth is not a platform for human life. It's a living being. We're not on it but part of it. Its health is our health." The spells and rituals that follow address the healing work we are called to do on behalf of Earth and ultimately our own sustainability as human beings.

RETURN TO MOTHER EARTH'S EMBRACE

PURPOSE OF SPELL: Has it been too long since you have connected to our planet? This outdoor ritual will cleanse you of any energy blockages and reunite your energy with Mother Earth.

SUGGESTED TIMING:
Rainy night

ITEMS NEEDED:

- Jar (empty pickle jar will work well)
- Twine

MAGICKAL INGREDIENTS:

- 1 stalk of thyme
- 1 stalk of rosemary
- 1 stalk of parsley
- 1 clear quartz crystal

SPELLWORK

✦ Place your empty jar outside with the clear quartz crystal in the center. Leave the jar out overnight on a rainy night to collect rainwater from Mother Earth.

✦ The next day, when the rain has stopped and the sun is shining, prepare for the ritual by tying the three stalks of herbs together at their base. Use three knots to secure the twine. Retrieve your jar of magickally charged rainwater.

✦ Head to an outdoor location with your jar and herb bundle. Perhaps you have already designated a sacred space outside for yourself. Perhaps you can find a location that inspires you. Walk the location barefoot. Feel the muddy earth squishing between your toes. Notice how the mud clings to you, hugging you, and welcoming you. Ground and center yourself in Mother Earth's presence. Take deep breaths of the air. Appreciate the scenery. Feel gratitude.

✦ Now, grasp your herb bundle and dip the tips of the herbs into the rainwater and incant:

"In gratitude and in awe of Mother Nature's gifts,
This herbal bundle of earthly goodness to the sky I lift."

✦ Lift the bundle to the sun with an outstretched arm. Feel the warmth of the sun sending loving rays down to the bundle and your person. Feel drops of the rainwater falling off the bundle and blessing your face.

✦ Dip your bundle back in the rainwater. Now lower your bundle and asperge it in all four directions and say:

"North, south, east, and west
I am a child of Earth
North, south, east, and west
I am a lover of Earth
North, south, east, and west
I am a protector of Earth.
As I am and so it will be, from now until eternity."

✦ Seal the ritual and your loving intent by burying the piece of clear quartz at the sacred location. Pour the remaining rainwater over the buried quartz to compact the earth and nourish the quartz energy. Leave the bundle of herbs tied to a branch or bush as a gift to Mother Earth. You are now healed of any disconnect from Mother Earth.

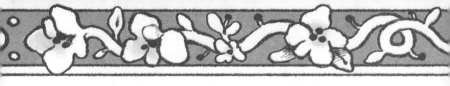

HEALING HUMAN APATHY

PURPOSE OF SPELL: This ritual incantation uses the power of fire and blade to ignite a call to action from all of Earth's citizens. This spell works to heal the apathy many feel about the health of our planet and encourages stewardship and protective action from humankind.

SUGGESTED TIMING:
Full moon

ITEMS NEEDED:

- 8 candles
- Lighter
- Athame

MAGICKAL INGREDIENTS:

- Citrine crystals
- Green aventurine crystals
- Jasper crystals
- Clear quartz crystals

SPELLWORK

✦ Arrange the eight candles in a line across your altar. Place the crystals between each candle to link the energies.

✦ Follow this incantation of hope:

> *"I light these four candles*
> *And call on the corners."*

Light the first four candles.

> *"I light the next four*
> *for Earth's sons and daughters."*

Light the next four candles.

> *"I draw my blade through each flame*
> *Left to right, slow and steady*
> *And call out to all humans*
> *'Hark now! At the ready!'"*

Draw your athame through all flames to encourage action.

✦ Now raise the cleansed blade high overhead:

> *"Rush off to the aid of our Earth that needs healing!*
> *Thus I raise my athame strong to the ceiling.*
> *The call to action is heard far and wide*
> *This planet will heal with the help of all humankind."*

✦ Feel the energy flow from your heart, up your arm, and out the blade, and shower down on humankind. Stand poised as a fountain of strength, working on behalf of Mother Earth to inspire healing stewardship across the globe.

MAGICK FOR THE ANIMALS

PURPOSE OF SPELL: This spell protects animals and wildlife from threats to their health and growth by channeling healing, flourishing energy from the power of rain and Mother Earth.

SUGGESTED TIMING:
Just before it rains

ITEMS NEEDED:
- Chalk
- Pavement or a chalkboard

MAGICKAL INGREDIENTS:
- Clear quartz crystals
- Green aventurine crystals

SPELLWORK

✦ Identify three to five animals, especially any on an endangered species list, that you would like to send healing energy to. Look up their likeness for your reference.

✦ Draw on the pavement or chalkboard the likeness of these animals. Don't worry about artistic talent. This is about drawing the animals with love and care. Your intention is to draw healing vibes.

✦ In their eyes, place the quartz and aventurine crystals to link earthly positive energies to the animal likenesses and thus the animals themselves.

✦ When finished, hold your hands out over your artwork and incant:

"Blessed Mother, come hither with rain
Protect these animals, heal their pain."

✦ Leave the drawings and crystals outside to be washed clean by the power of rain. Know Mother Earth has heard your prayer, collected your magick, and afforded the animals renewed protection.

✦ Collect the crystals and place them in a bowl near a sunny window to keep the magick energy flowing out to wildlife. Repeat the process as you feel is needed.

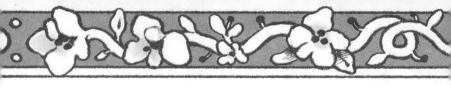

TREE HUGGER CHARM

PURPOSE OF SPELL: This charm seeks to restore and bolster the health and abundance of the worldwide tree population. Work with the natural elements of local trees to send deep-rooted healing to all of Earth's trees.

SUGGESTED TIMING:
Waxing moon, full moon

ITEMS NEEDED:

- Sturdy, dry branch, fallen from a local tree, at least a foot in length
- Athame
- Leaves, nuts, bark, fruit, or pine cones from various local trees

ITEMS CONT.

- Ribbon or twine

MAGICKAL INGREDIENTS:

- Jasper crystals
- Clear quartz crystals
- Cedar oil (as needed)
- Eucalyptus oil (as needed)

SPELLWORK

✦ Engrave a pentagram on one side of your branch and Earth's symbol on the other side of the branch.

✦ Seal the magick of these symbols by anointing the pentagram with eucalyptus oil and Earth's symbol with cedar oil.

✦ Tie the ends of the ribbon on either end of the stick, leaving enough slack to hang the branch comfortably from a hook or nail in your wall.

✦ Next, adorn the branch with trinkets by tying your locally foraged tree ingredients and crystals with ribbon so that they hang down from the branch.

✦ Hang your branch so it is level across your wall. You may choose an indoor location, or perhaps you prefer this charm to hang on your porch or patio so it may blow in the wind. Your charm is a labor of healing love, emanating growth and sustainability to the worldwide tree population.

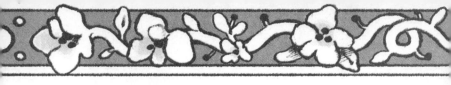

EARTH'S BOUNTY RENEWED

PURPOSE OF SPELL: Use this ritual blessing to infuse loving growth to the world's food supply and help heal regions affected by food insecurity.

SUGGESTED TIMING:
New moon

ITEMS NEEDED:
- Bowl of warm water
- Athame

MAGICKAL INGREDIENTS:
- Stalk of parsley
- 1 teaspoon garlic powder
- 1 teaspoon ginger powder
- Green aventurine crystals
- Citrine crystals

SPELLWORK

✦ Add the spices and crystals to your bowl of warm water. Use your athame to stir the mixture deosil three times to charge it.

✦ Stand in front of your houseplants, vegetable garden, or favorite outdoor plant with your parsley stalk and bowl of magick healing water. Dip the parsley stalk in the water and asperge your plant seven times.

✦ As you asperge, incant:

"Magick rain of garlic and ginger,
Banish frailty, let weakness not linger.
By power of my craft I dowse this potion,
In loving growth and devotion.

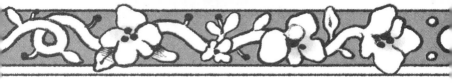

Worldwide crops grow fruitful and tall,
To nourish our brethren with food for all."

✦ Discard any remaining water mixture outdoors on a patch of dirt. Leave your crystals outside overnight or on a windowsill to emanate the magick of the spell to the land.

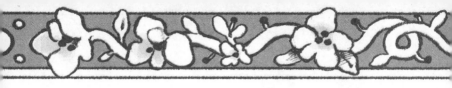

WATER CLEAN AND CLEAR

PURPOSE OF SPELL: This kitchen witch spell serves as a potion to help heal drinking water impurities and promote clean, drinkable water for all.

SUGGESTED TIMING:
Full moon

ITEMS NEEDED:

- Saucepan with cover
- Cheesecloth

ITEMS CONT.

- Large jar
- 1 sliced lemon

MAGICKAL INGREDIENTS:

- 3 sprigs of fresh mint
- 1 cup fresh sage leaves or ¼ cup dried

SPELLWORK

✦ Fill your saucepan with 3 cups of water. Heat it over high heat and bring to a rapid boil.

✦ Drop the mint into the boiling water and say:

"Mint, work your protective magick."

✦ Drop the lemon slices into the boiling water and say:

"Lemon, work your cleansing magick."

✦ Drop the sage leaves into the boiling water and say:

"Sage, work your healing magick."

THE HEALING POWER OF WITCHCRAFT

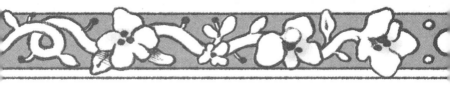

✦ Reduce the heat to simmer. Let the mixture reduce and steam for an hour or so as the magickal properties combine. When ready, take the mixture off the stove, strain the herbs and lemon out through a cheesecloth, and let the water cool. Discard or compost the herbs and lemon.

✦ Pour the cooled water into a jar and leave it to charge under the full moon. The next day, bring the magick water to a local running water source, or use your sink drain if that is not possible. Pour the magickal water out into the flowing water or down the drain and know its cleansing, healing power is now dispersed into the fresh waters of our planet.

AIR CLEAN AND CLEAR

PURPOSE OF SPELL: This spell uses the power of smoke to cleanse the air and send healing air energy worldwide.

SUGGESTED TIMING:
Waning moon, new moon

ITEMS NEEDED:

- Lighter
- Ashtray
- Twine

ITEMS CONT.

- Cookie sheet

MAGICKAL INGREDIENTS:

- Bundle of dried sage, oregano, and rosemary
- 3 drops lavender oil

SPELLWORK

✦ Create the bundle by securing together fresh sage, oregano, and rosemary stalks in stick form with twine. Wrap the twine around the herbs tightly, as the herbs will shrink in the drying process. Charge your bundle by adding three drops of lavender to the tip and making a pentagram with your finger on the bundle.

✦ Heat your oven to 180°F. Place the bundle on a cookie sheet and bake in the oven for 2 hours. Adjust time if needed. Once fully dried, remove the bundle from the oven and let it cool. Snip the twine off completely, as your bundle should now be compacted by the drying process. Handle the bundle delicately since dried herbs are brittle.

✦ Head to your favorite room in your home. This should be a place you feel inspired, comfortable, and safe. Make sure there is a bit of free floor space for you to maneuver. Open all the windows in the room and let the fresh air pour in. Feel that air meet the warm energy of your home and your healing intention you set by creating the magickal herb bundle.

✦ Play some meditation music if you desire. Center yourself with a meditation on the lightness of the joy and wholeness. Light the bundle. Slowly walk in a circle, deosil, around the room with the lit bundle in one hand. Hold an ashtray under the bundle to catch any stray embers. Keep the lighter nearby in case the bundle goes out and you need to relight it. This is common, especially if you move a bit too fast. Simply relight the bundle and relight your intention.

✦ As you walk, make figure eights with your burning bundle. Eight is the number of transformations. Notice how the burning herbs transform the room with a dualistic quality of smoky lightness and an earthy aroma of grounding. Lean into this powerful energy, and send your healing intentions out the windows with your full strength. As the air and smells float out your windows, so will the earth's air quality transform and improve. Burn the bundle completely. Once it's out, shut your windows to send the energy on its healing way.

PROTECTING THE WILD OUTDOORS

PURPOSE OF SPELL: Humankind honors and protects Mother Earth by designating natural wonders as national parks and wildlife preserves. This ritual uses creative process energy, creatrix witchcraft, to send healthful and wholeful vibes to protect our most sacred natural wonders and spaces.

SUGGESTED TIMING:
Full moon

ITEMS NEEDED:

- Poster board
- Photos from magazines or printed pictures of natural wonders that resonate with you

ITEMS CONT.

- Scotch tape
- Marker
- Cotton swab

MAGICKAL INGREDIENTS:

- 4 fresh mint leaves
- Ylang-ylang oil

SPELLWORK

✦ Begin by drawing Earth's symbol in the center of the poster board. Draw the symbols for the four elements, one in each corner. Dab a small amount of ylang-ylang on your cotton swab and seal the protective, healing intent of the symbols by tracing them with the oil.

✦ Arrange your collage of natural beauty. Inspire yourself with the wonders we are so lucky to behold. Feel gratitude for Earth's bounty. Secure the pictures to the board with tape, saying the name of the location in the picture as you do.

✦ Place your finished creation under the light of the full moon. Seal it by placing one of the four mint leaves on each of the elemental symbols. The next morning, hang the picture somewhere meaningful to you in your home. Use the mint leaves in your morning tea, hot chocolate, coffee, or iced water to carry this healing, protective intention with you into the world.

SALT OF THE SEVEN CONTINENTS

PURPOSE OF SPELL: This spell unites the seven continents, and all their inhabitants, in a protective, healing, green salt potion.

SUGGESTED TIMING:
Full moon

MAGICKAL INGREDIENTS:
- 7 dried bay leaves

ITEMS NEEDED:
- Mortar and pestle
- Black ink
- ½ cup salt

SPELLWORK

✦ On each bay leaf, write the name of one of the continents: North America, South America, Asia, Australia, Africa, Antarctica, Europe.

✦ Crumble the seven bay leaves into your mortar and add the salt.

✦ Grind the bay leaves and salt together for 10 to 15 minutes. This is labor. This is the work of drawing different elements together. This is a loving, healing result. Earth gives us all the magickal tools we need to heal and make positive changes, so let us bind together every land in supportive unity.

✦ The green salt becomes ready once it is fine and fully green, synthesized together in healing energy.

✦ Hold your tired hands over the mixture, palms down, and incant:

"By toil, by labor, in the name of world unity,
Hath created green salt for healing modality.
Spring forth from the earth a new order of compassion
Let us join together on a mission, a healed world we will fashion."

✦ Use your green salt in magickal workings for healing and protecting Earth's natural resources and inhabitants with the power of the seven continents at your aid.

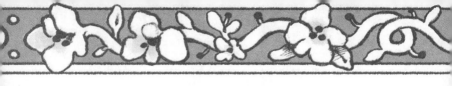

OCEANS BLUE

PURPOSE OF SPELL: This spell casts healing energy worldwide to all five oceans and their inhabitants.

SUGGESTED TIMING:
Waxing moon, full moon

ITEMS NEEDED:

- 5 small jars or bowls
- 1 empty fishbowl, water pitcher, flower vase, or other large glass container

ITEMS CONT.

- 2 cups water
- Blue ribbon

MAGICKAL INGREDIENTS:

- 1 sprig of rosemary
- 1 fluorite crystal
- 5 drops frankincense oil

SPELLWORK

✦ Disperse the 2 cups of water evenly among the five small bowls or jars.

✦ Place one drop of oil into each bowl. As you do so, state the name of each ocean—Pacific, Atlantic, Indian, Southern, Arctic—to summon their attention.

✦ Drop the fluorite into the center of the large empty glass container. One at a time, pour each bowl of water into the large container, speaking the ocean names again. As you pour each one, watch the waters unite while the healing fluorite touches them all. Understand how all our oceans are connected and all are relying on the power of the individual to heal.

✦ Tie the ribbon tightly around the top of the container's rim. Make five knots to seal the ribbon, again incanting the name of each ocean as you do.

✦ Finally, seal the healing intent of the mixture by drawing a pentagram shape in the water five times with the sprig of rosemary. Set the bowl near a sunny window and keep it out until evaporated. The magickal energy you created has returned to the sky to rain down upon Earth's oceans with healing power.

HEAL EARTH FROM FLOODING

PURPOSE OF SPELL: This spell helps to stem the tide of harmful floodwaters and heal the affected Earth back to balance.

SUGGESTED TIMING:
Full moon, waning moon

ITEMS NEEDED:

- Bowl of dry soil
- Athame
- Bowl of water
- Large sponge

MAGICKAL INGREDIENTS:

- ½ teaspoon garlic powder
- ½ teaspoon turmeric powder
- 3 drops peppermint oil
- 3 drops eucalyptus oil

SPELLWORK

✦ Mix the garlic and turmeric into the soil with your athame by stirring deosil seven times.

✦ Mix the oils into your water with your athame by stirring deosil seven times.

✦ Submerge your sponge into the magick water. As you do, meditate on drawing away the water.

✦ Transfer it over the bowl of magick soil and squeeze all the water out onto the soil. Meditate on receptivity of the earth to water. Repeat this process seven times.

✦ Spread the soil over your houseplants and garden or keep it in a jar to spread healing, receptive energy to flood-ridden locations.

HEAL EARTH FROM WILDFIRE

PURPOSE OF SPELL: This spell invokes the power of water, earth, and human action to calm wildfires and heal flame-ravaged Earth.

SUGGESTED TIMING:
New moon, waxing moon

ITEMS NEEDED:

- 3 candles
- Lighter
- Small bowl of water

ITEMS CONT.

- Small bowl of salt or soil
- Empty jar with lid

MAGICKAL INGREDIENTS:

- ½ teaspoon chamomile
- Smoky quartz crystals

SPELLWORK

✦ Line up the three candles across your altar horizontally.

✦ Place the bowl of water in front of the first candle, the bowl of salt in front of the middle candle, and the empty jar with a lid in front of the third candle.

✦ Center yourself and tap into the energy of the wildfire by lighting the candles one at a time.

✦ Extinguish the first candle by plunging the flame into the bowl of water and incanting:

"May healing waters fall, and healing waters flow,
Put out the fire, penetrate the earth, new flora will you sow."

CONTINUED >>>

✦ Extinguish the second candle by smothering the flame into the salt and incanting:

"May Earth withstand the burning flame,
Rejuvenate the scorched plains,
Heal the forests, calm the jungles,
Spring forth renewal from the remains."

✦ Pour the salt and water into the empty jar. Add the chamomile and smoky quartz to the jar.

✦ Extinguish the third candle by blowing it out with your breath. Catch the smoke in the jar of salt and water and quickly close the lid. Incant:

"As my breath did snuff the dancing blaze,
Let human action lead the way
We band together to bring healing to our Mother Earth,
So it is, done as we say."

✦ Swirl the contents of the jar three times and set it out under the full moon to fully charge. In the morning, discard the jar's contents back to the earth. Place the crystal in a fresh bowl of water for a bit to cleanse the energy it absorbed in healing the earth from wildfire.

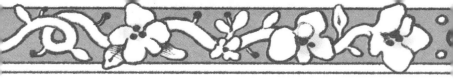

HEAL EARTH FROM DROUGHT

PURPOSE OF SPELL: This spell helps heal areas of Earth affected by drought.

SUGGESTED TIMING:
Waxing moon

ITEMS NEEDED:
- Sphere-shaped rock or clear quartz crystal
- Small bowl

MAGICKAL INGREDIENTS:
- ½ cup dried chamomile
- 3 drops bergamot oil

SPELLWORK

✦ Start this spell during the waxing moon period.

✦ Place your chamomile in the small bowl. With your finger, draw the water symbol in the herb to charge its water properties to the forefront.

✦ Select your spherical rock or clear quartz crystal to represent Earth.

CONTINUED >>>

✦ Hold it in your hands gently, cupping it in a closed fashion, and say:

> *"Mother Earth, you are suffering from thirst*
> *I impart you healing love to bear the worst.*
> *Send healing rains to your parched plains*
> *Your ground refreshed, your fauna nursed."*

✦ Place the rock in the chamomile bowl and cover it with the chamomile. Anoint the mixture with three drops of bergamot oil to seal the water-drawing intention. Let the bowl sit by a moonlit window until the night of the full moon.

✦ During the full moon, take the rock out of its bed of chamomile and bring it to running water. Throw the rock in running water and let the water carry its energy to the drought-afflicted region. If an ocean, lake, brook, or stream is not readily accessible for you, throwing the rock down a storm drain or washing it out of your yard with a garden hose will work just as well. The intention is to let the power of water you have manifested be sent on its healing way.

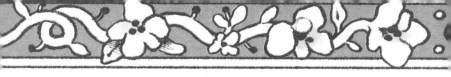

PLANET PUMPKIN CHARM

PURPOSE OF SPELL: Create this charm as a beacon of healing light for planet Earth.

SUGGESTED TIMING:
Full moon, Samhain

ITEMS CONT.

- Lighter

ITEMS NEEDED:

- Athame or carving knife
- Pumpkin
- Candle

MAGICKAL INGREDIENTS:

- Green aventurine crystals
- Cedar oil (as needed)

SPELLWORK

✦ Cut open the pumpkin by carving a circle around the stem and pulling on the stem to remove. Clean the inside of the top and set the top aside. Scoop out all insides of the pumpkin and add to your compost. As you do so, envision the pumpkin as planet Earth; your intent is to clear away any energy blocking Earth from healing.

✦ Carve healing symbols into your pumpkin. Perhaps you carve the symbol for Earth. Maybe you prefer a pentagram, a heart, or a sigil you create yourself. Get lovingly creative!

CONTINUED >>>

✦ Once finished carving your healing symbols, anoint your candle with the healing cedar oil and place it in the center of the pumpkin. Surround the candle with green aventurine.

✦ When ready, light your candle, place the top back on your pumpkin, and incant:

> *"Fruit from the earth, round, and bright*
> *Serve my plea for your Mother tonight.*
> *Carved and dressed with love and care*
> *Your light sends healing everywhere*
> *From east to west, north to south,*
> *From mountaintop to river mouth.*
> *From canyons deep to oceans wide,*
> *Your healing light does now abide."*

✦ Your jack-o'-lantern shines bright, healing light across the world.

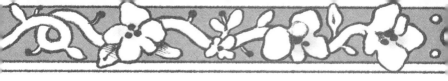

GROUP SPELL TO HEAL EARTH

PURPOSE OF SPELL: This spell uses the powerful energy of a devoted group to raise healing energy for Mother Earth.

SUGGESTED TIMING:
Full moon

ITEMS NEEDED:

- Large apple
- Bowl and small spoon
- Apple peeler
- Athame

ITEMS CONT.

- 7 candles
- Lighter

MAGICKAL INGREDIENTS:

- 2 tablespoons cinnamon
- 1 green aventurine crystal
- 1 clear quartz crystal

SPELLWORK

✦ Gather all group members around a table.

✦ Place the bowl in the center of the table. Add the cinnamon to the bowl. Place the apple on top. Lay the crystals on either side of the apple. Encircle the bowl with the seven candles.

✦ Once this is set up, the leader should call for quiet and centering focus on the apple in the bowl. The leader should note the apple represents Earth, the cinnamon is for grounding and spell success, and the crystals are for green healing.

CONTINUED >>>

LEADER:

"Seven candles are with us tonight, seven candles we shall light,
Our magick sent to seven continents,
Flora and fauna, all inhabitants.
Our magick flows to the seven seas,
Marine habitats, we call to thee."

Leader lights the seven candles.

LEADER:

"Healing energy is now invoked,
These healing flames we now stoke
Burn strong and bright, reach planet wide,
In healing devotion our spell abides."

Leader picks up the apple from the bowl.

LEADER:

"Apple round and salubrious, you represent the earth to us.
We hold you close with hands of care,
Please send healing love everywhere."

Leader holds the apple close to their heart and then passes the apple to the next participant.

✦ The next participant holds the apple close to their heart and repeats the incantation:

"Apple round and salubrious, you represent the earth to us,
We hold you close with hands of care,
Please send healing love everywhere."

✦ Repeat for every participant.

✦ When the apple reaches the leader again, the leader holds the apple high and says:

"By power of this group's will, we release the earth from all ills."

✦ Leader peels the skin off the apple to shed negative energy.

✦ Leader cuts the apple into as many slices as there are participants and gives one slice to each person.

✦ Participants may add a little cinnamon to the apple from the bowl via the spoon if they desire.

LEADER:
*"Now together we do eat, the apple powerful and sweet,
We appreciate this gift of Earth, we honor Mother Nature's worth.
Far and wide, from forest to sea,
We heal our planet, so mote it be."*

ALL:
"So mote it be."

✦ All eat the apple to seal the spell for earthly healing.

✦ By the power of the group's will, magickal healing is dispersed far and wide, creating lasting, positive change.

CLOSING THOUGHTS

Healing witchcraft is a beautiful, loving process, worthy of lifelong devotion. My hope is you may return to this text again and again as healing challenges arise. Healing witchcraft is also deeply personal and profoundly impactful. Use these spells as the foundation with which to weave and profess your own, unique style of changing the world. The more authentic the witch's working, the more powerful the result, so let us step boldly into our healing power and proudly create healing magick. Let us go forth and live the magick we create.

GLOSSARY

Witchcraft comes with its own way of describing and naming things. Here are a few terms common to witchcraft that you will encounter in this book and their meanings.

AMULET: An object worn or carried by a person to draw good luck or a specific energy to them.

ANOINT: To apply ritual oil.

ASPERGE: To sprinkle liquid with magickal intent.

ATHAME: A ritual knife.

BOOK OF SHADOWS: A witch's collection of personal magickal workings and knowledge.

CALLING QUARTERS: A ritual at the start of spellwork invoking the four directions and elements.

CHAKRAS: A Sanskrit term referring to the seven energy centers within the human body.

CHALICE: A ceremonial cup, representative of the element water.

CHARGING: The process of bringing an item, particularly crystals, to full power after magickal creation or use.

CHARMS: Objects, or a group of objects, that correspond to drawing a certain energy. Charms attract the energy of their contents.

CORRESPONDENCES: A metaphysical property of an object that holds the same energy as the intention of the magickal workings at hand.

CREATRIX WITCHCRAFT: The practice of creating art or crafting goods as the mode of spellwork.

DEOSIL: Clockwise.

GRIMOIRE: A book of general witchcraft knowledge, often handed down through generations.

GROUNDING (ALSO CALLED CENTERING): A calming process meant to connect our minds with our bodies and the earth.

INCANTATION: Predetermined words uttered during a spell or as a spell for magickal force.

INTENTION: Focused willpower toward an identified outcome.

MORTAR AND PESTLE: A bowl (mortar) and blunted instrument (pestle) used to grind plants and herbs.

PENTAGRAM: Five-pointed star representing the four elements and spirit, drawn in divine proportion.

POPPET: An image or a doll used to represent another person in spellwork.

POTION: A concoction intentionally crafted with magickal ingredients to bring about change.

PRAXIS: Practice as distinguished from theory, yielding wisdom in addition to knowledge.

RITUAL: A premeditated set of magickal steps honoring or inviting a chosen energy, meant to align, cleanse, and enhance rather than change or transform.

SACHET: A small bag of herbs or other magickal tools used to draw energy.

SIGIL: A symbol drawn to represent an entity or an idea for magickal use.

SPELL CASTING: Intentional magick; manipulating or channeling energy as a means to an end using specific steps and methods.

SYMPATHY MAGICK: Magick performed on behalf of another person or entity.

THIRD EYE: A term for the pineal gland, located in the forehead, a locus of intuition and perception beyond the ordinary.

WHEEL OF THE YEAR: Eight sabbats (holidays) that make up the pagan calendar.

WIDDERSHINS: Counterclockwise.

WORTCUNNING/ CUNNING: Knowledge and use of plants in healing.

RESOURCES

BIRTH CHART: You may access a free birth chart calculator and corresponding book suggestions at witchwithme.com/birth-chart.

MYERS–BRIGGS TEST may be found at Myersbriggs.org.

ENNEAGRAM TEST may be found at EnneagramInstitute.com.

INDEX

A

Achievements, celebrating, 194–195
Addiction, recovering from, 167–168
Air, 22, 36
Allspice (*Pimenta officinalis*), 30
  in easing anxieties of loved ones, 153
  emanating into cooking, 232
Altar, 38
  creating display to summon confidence and courage, 137
  location of, 21–22
  surface of, 22
Amethyst, 32
  in alignment of mind and body, 130, 131
  in being accepted for authentic identities, 163, 164
  in casting off moon cycle disappointments, 192
  in creating moon water elixir, 66, 67
  in creation of home sanctuary, 227, 228
  in disconnecting with universe, 115, 116
  in foot soak in summoning forgiveness, 133
  in getting better sleep, 72
  in healing self-doubt, 190
  in healing weakness in psychic abilities, 119, 120
  in improving memory, 92
  in shining protective energy into home, 215, 216
Amulet, 269
Anger, 78
  assuaging, 83–84
Animals
  protecting from threats, 240–241
  relationship with yourself, 17
Anise (*Pimpinella anisum*), 30
  in drawing calming vibes to the anxious mind, 81
Anointing, 35, 267
Apathy, 78
  healing, 238–239

Apples
  in clearing body of energy that dampens longevity, 156–157
  in raising healing energy for Earth, 263–265
Aquarius, 13
Aries, 12, 13
Artistic pursuits, 9
Asperging, 36, 267
Astrological birth chart calculator, 8–9
Athame, 267
  defined, 27
  in disconnecting with universe, 115
  in easing anxieties of your loved ones, 153
  in healing apathy, 238, 239
  in healing common cold, 71
  in healing from negative, toxic patterns, 98, 99
  in healing negative responses, 123
  in healing regions affected by food security, 244
  in maintaining nutrition, 54
  in raising healing energy for Earth, 263–265
  in recovering from addiction, 167
  in repairing friendships, 161
Authentic identities, being accepted for, 163–164
Authentic self, revealing your most, 56–57

B

Baking soda, in renewing heart to possibility of love, 111
Balance, grounding and finding, 79–80
Ball of energy method, 40
Basil (*Ocimum basilicum*), 28
  emanating into cooking, 232
  in harnessing healing power of, 225, 226
  in healing energy interference, 196
  in healing "lone wolf" attitudes, 188
  prior to lovemaking, 68
Basil oil, 33
  in healing self-doubt, 165
  in infusing energy of love and healing, 171

Bay leaves (*Laurus nobilis*), 29
  emanating into cooking, 232
  in getting past being stuck in the past, 169, 170
  in giving magickal protection to spirit, 121
  in healing indifference, 182, 183
  in releasing hope, 135–136
  in releasing pessimism, 233–234
  in sachet in recovering from surgery, 149
  in soothing spirit, 219, 220
  in summoning confidence and courage, 137
  in unification of continents, 252
Bells, 34
  in creating witchy bell charm, 209
  in creating witchy charm, 209–210
  in healing negative responses, 123
Beltane, 10–11
Bergamot oil, 34
  for body positivity, 76
  in celebrating achievements, 194
  in connecting group with healing prayers, 202
  in healing Earth from drought, 259
  in healing self-doubt, 165
  in healing weakness in psychic abilities, 119, 120
  in lifting depression, 85
  in reducing stress, 87
  in renewing spirit from negative energies, 139
  in struggling with mental health, 159
Birth chart, 268
  astrological calculator for, 8–9
Black pepper (*Piper nigrum*), 30
  in making healing poppets, 147
  in release from jealousy, 108, 109
Black salt, creation of, in healing negative energy, 223–224

Body
    alignment with mind,
        130–132
    healing of, 46–77
    positivity and, 76–77
    recharging and renewing
        your, 74–75
Book of Shadows, 175, 267
Bradbury, Ray, 5
Broken heart, healing of,
    89–91

C

Cairns, magic of, 79–80
Calling corners, 39
Calling quarters, 39, 267
Calming vibes, drawing to the
    anxious mind, 81–82
Camaraderie, bringing into
    home, 221–222
Cancer, 13
Candle lighting
    in alleviating effects of
        imposter syndrome,
        100–101
    in assuaging anger, 83–84
    in beating fatigue, 52
    in being accepted for
        authentic identities,
        163–164
    in casting off moon cycle
        disappointments, 192
    in charging your crystals,
        47
    in connecting group
        with healing prayers,
        202–203
    in creating happy and
        optimistic energy,
        94–95
    in fostering patience,
        106–107
    in healing apathy, 238–239
    in healing Earth from
        wildfire, 257–258
    in healing from grief,
        154–155
    in healing from negative,
        toxic patterns, 98–99
    in healing from spiritual
        rut, 126–127
    in healing indifference,
        182–183
    in healing low energy,
        178–179
    in healing negative
        responses, 123–125
    in healing self-doubt,
        165–166, 190–191

in improving memory, 92
prior to lovemaking, 69
in raising healing energy
    for Earth, 263–265
in recharging your body,
    74–75
in renewing heart to
    possibility of, 111–112
in repairing friendships,
    161–162
in soothing spirit, 219–220
in struggling with mental
    health, 159–160
Candles, 22
    dressing, 35
Capricorn, 13
Carnelian, 32
    in aiding conception, 60
    in alignment of mind and
        body, 130, 131, 132
    in being accepted for
        authentic identities,
        163, 164
    in celebrating
        achievements, 194
    in charging your crystals,
        47, 48
    in combating lethargic
        effects, 158
    in creating happy and
        optimistic energy, 94
    in creating sigils, 174
    in drawing strength to
        work, 217
    in healing from spiritual
        rut, 126
    prior to lovemaking, 68
    in recovering from
        addiction, 158, 167
    in shining protective
        energy into home,
        215, 216
Carrier oil, 33
Casting a circle, 38–39
Cauldron, 11, 27
Cayenne pepper (Capsicum
    annuum), 30
    in getting past being stuck
        in the past, 169, 170
    in healing common cold,
        70
    in healing indifference, 182
    in maintaining better
        nutrition, 44, 54
Cedar oil, 34
    in boosting your healing
        strength, 96
    in creating cohesion
        between groups and
        community, 200

in creating witchy bell
    charm, 209
emanating into cooking,
    232
in healing light for Earth,
    261, 262
in helping committed
    relationships through
    rough patches, 151
in maintaining better
    nutrition, 54, 55
in recovering from
    addiction, 167
in restoring trees, 242
in shining protective
    energy into home, 215
in summoning confidence
    and courage, 137
Cedarwood oil
    in enhancing receptivity
        to psychic messages,
        117–118
    prior to lovemaking, 68
Centering, 20, 34, 267
Chakras, 22, 130, 267
Chalice, 22, 267
Chamomile (Chamaemelum
    nobile), 29
    in assuaging anger, 83, 84
    in creating happy and
        optimistic energy, 94
    in foot soak in summoning
        forgiveness, 133
    in healing discord, 176
    in healing Earth from
        drought, 259
    in healing Earth from
        wildfire, 257, 258
    in struggling with mental
        health, 159
Change, healing negative
    responses to, 123–125
Charging, 267
Charms, 23, 267
Cinnamon (Cinnamomum
    verum), 30
    in bringing joy into home,
        221, 222
    in clearing body of energy
        that dampens longevity,
        156, 157
    in foot soak in summoning
        forgiveness, 133
    in healing common cold,
        70
    in improving
        concentration, 102
    in improving memory, 92
    prior to lovemaking, 68, 69

in raising healing energy
for Earth, 263, 265
in reducing stress, 87
Circle
casting a, 38–39
closing the, 41
Citrine, 32
in alignment of mind and
body, 130, 131
in alleviating effects of
imposter syndrome,
100–101
in being accepted for
authentic identities,
163, 164
in building a witch's ladder,
230
in charging your crystals,
47, 48
in combating lethargic
effects, 158
in creating happy and
optimistic energy, 94
in creating sigils, 174
in drawing strength to
work, 217
in healing apathy, 238
in healing from spiritual
rut, 126
in healing home of clutter,
213
in healing regions affected
by food security, 244
in healing righteousness,
141
in healing self-doubt, 165,
190
in maintaining better
nutrition, 54
prior to lovemaking, 68
in renewing spirit from
negative energies, 139
in summoning confidence
and courage, 137
Clear quartz, 27
in aiding conception, 60
in alignment of mind and
body, 130, 132
in alleviating effects of
imposter syndrome,
100–101
in being accepted for
authentic identities,
163, 164
in being proactive about
negative energy, 218
in building a witch's ladder,
229, 231
in cleansing energy
blockages, 236

in combating lethargic
effects, 158
in creating moon water
elixir, 66, 67
in disconnecting with
universe, 115
in giving magickal
protection to spirit, 121
in healing apathy, 238
in healing discord, 176
in healing ego weaknesses,
180
in healing feelings of
isolation, 198
in healing from grief, 154
in healing righteousness,
141, 142
in healing weakness in
psychic abilities, 119, 120
in improving memory, 92
in protecting against
injustice, 184
in protecting animals, 240
in raising healing energy
for Earth, 263
in relieving tension
headaches, 62, 63
in restoring trees, 242
in revealing authentic
self, 56
in struggling with mental
health, 159
Closing the circle, 41
Clove (*Syzygium
aromaticum*), 30
in aiding conception, 60
in being proactive about
negative energy, 218
in dispersing negative
energies, 150
in drawing calming vibes
to the anxious mind, 81
in easing anxieties of loved
ones, 153
in healing from negative,
toxic patterns, 98–99
in improving memory, 92
in reducing stress, 87
in release from jealousy,
108
Clutter, healing home of,
213–214
Coconut oil, in renewing heart
to possibility of, 111
Commitment
helping relationships
through rough patches,
151–152
to knowledge and learning,
15

Common cold, healing, 70–71
Community
creating cohesion between
groups and, 200–201
healing your, 144–203
Concentration, improving,
102–103
Conception, 60–61
Connection
to the cosmos, 12–15
to nature, 9–12
to self, 8–9
Containers, 27
Continents, unification of,
252–253
Cooking, 9
healing moon water elixir
and, 66, 67
infusing, with healing love,
232–233
moon healing for the
broken heart and, 90
Correspondences, 22–23, 267
Cosmic energy, aligning spells
with, 12
Cosmic witch, 19
Cosmos, connection to the,
12–15
Covens, 19–20
defined, 173
Creating, 9
Creatrix witchcraft, 267
Crystals, 31–32
charging your, 47–49
Cunning, 70, 268

D

Dancing
in disconnecting with
universe, 116
of flames, 69, 73, 123, 258
of sunlight, 132
Deosil motion, 47, 67, 267
Depression, lifting, 85–86
Diffusers, 33
Discord, healing of, 176–177
Doubt, 78
Dressing a candle, 35
Drought, healing Earth from,
259–260
Dualistic energy code,
following the, 17
Dumb Supper for the
grieving, 154–155

E

Earth, 9, 22, 36
  healing from drought,
    259–260
  healing from floods, 256
  healing light for, 261–262
  protecting from wildfire,
    257–258
  raising healing energy for,
    263–265
Eclectic witch, 19
Ego
  assuaging, 190–191
  healing weaknesses in,
    180–181
Elemental witch, 18
Elements, 22
  symbols for the, 36
Energy. *See also* Negative
    energy
  cleansing blockages,
    236–237
  creating happy and
    optimistic, 94–95
  getting boost of, 52–53
  healing interference,
    196–197
  healing low, 178–179
  raising, 40
  raising healing for Earth,
    263–265
  rebalancing, 41
Enjoy yourself, 40
Enneagram, 9
Enneagram test, 268
Epsom salt, in renewing heart
  to possibility of, 111
Essential oils, 33–34
  in beating fatigue, 52
  for body positivity, 76
  in boosting concentration,
    102–103
  in boosting energy, 52
  in celebrating
    achievements, 194–195
  in drawing strength to
    work, 217
  in healing common cold,
    70
  in healing home of clutter,
    213
  in healing self-doubt, 165
  in healing weakness in
    psychic abilities, 119–120
  in improving
    concentration, 102–103
  in lifting depression, 85
  prior to lovemaking, 68, 69
  in recovering from
    addiction, 167
  in reducing stress, 87
  in struggling with mental
    health, 159
  in summoning confidence
    and courage, 137
Eucalyptus oil, 34
  in combating lethargic
    effects, 158
  in healing common cold,
    70
  in healing Earth from
    floods, 256
  in healing home of clutter,
    213
  in healing low energy, 178
  in overcoming lingering
    illness, 64
  in restoring trees, 242

F

Family, healing your, 146–172
Fatigue, beating, 52–53
Fear, 78
Feminine life cycle, 74
Figure eights, making, in
  cleansing air, 249
Fire, 22, 36
First quarter moon, 14
Floods, healing Earth from,
  256
Fluorite, 32
  in being proactive about
    negative energy, 218
  in casting off moon cycle
    disappointments, 192
  in creation of home
    sanctuary, 227, 228
  in giving magickal
    protection to spirit, 121
  in healing broken heart,
    89, 91
  in healing from negative,
    toxic patterns, 98–99
  in healing oceans, 254
  in making healing poppets,
    147, 148
  in overcoming lingering
    illness, 64
  in repairing friendships, 161
Food insecurity, healing
  regions affected by,
    244–245
Forgiveness, magickal foot
  soak in summoning,
    133–134

Frankincense oil, 33
  in being proactive about
    negative energy, 218
  in creating witchy bell
    charm, 209
  in drawing strength to
    work, 217
  in healing oceans, 254
  in recovering from
    addiction, 167
  in renewing heart to
    possibility of, 111
  in shining protective
    energy into home, 215
  in summoning confidence
    and courage, 137
Friends, healing your, 146–172
Friendship, repairing, 161–162
Full moon, 15
  in healing broken heart,
    90–91

G

Garlic (*Allium sativum*), 30
  in drawing pain from body,
    58, 59
  in healing common cold,
    70
  in healing Earth from
    floods, 256
  in healing from grief, 154
  in healing regions affected
    by food security, 244
Gemini, 13
Ginger (*Zingiber officinale*),
  30
  in healing common cold,
    70
  in healing negative
    energies, 211
  in healing regions affected
    by food security, 244
  in recharging your body,
    74
Glamour witch, 19
Goddess archetype, 74
Gossip, release from petty,
  108–109
Green aventurine, 32
  in alignment of mind and
    body, 130, 131
  in being accepted for
    authentic identities,
    163, 164
  for body positivity, 76
  in creating moon water
    elixir, 66
  in dispersing negative
    energies, 150

THE HEALING POWER OF WITCHCRAFT

in drawing strength to
work, 217
in harnessing healing
power of, 225, 226
in healing apathy, 238
in healing energy
interference, 196
in healing light for Earth,
261, 262
in healing "lone wolf"
attitudes, 188
in healing regions affected
by food security, 244
in healing self-doubt, 190
in maintaining better
nutrition, 54
in protecting animals, 240
in raising healing energy
for Earth, 263
in sachet in recovering
from surgery, 149
in shining protective
energy into home, 215
Green salt, in unification of
continents, 252–253
Green witch, 19
Grimoire, 20, 267
Grounding, 267
magickal tool of, 38–39
Groups
creating cohesion between
community and,
200–201
healing, 173–203
Guilt, healing spirit from
burden of, 128–129

H

Hashtags, exploring on
Instagram, 20
Hate, 78
Headaches, relieving tension,
62–63
Healed body, 45
Healed mind, 45
Healed spirit, 45, 110
Healing
harnessing power of, 7–24
of the planet, 235–265
preparing for work in,
25–42
of your body, 46–77
of your community,
144–203
of your friends and family,
146–172
of your groups, 173–203
of your home, 206–234
of your mind, 78–109

of your spirit, 110–142
of your world, 204–265
Healing Moon Water Elixir,
66–67, 139
Healing prayers, connecting
group with, 202–203
Healing vibes, emanating into
cooking, 232
Healing work, 45
preparing for, 25–77
setting the stage for, 37–42
Hearth witch, 19
Heavens, 9
Hedge witch, 19
Herbalism, 27
Herbs, 27–29
Home, healing of your,
206–234
Honey, in healing common
cold, 70, 71
Hope, releasing, 135–136
Household items, 34–35

I

Illness
overcoming lingering,
64–65
prevention of, 50–51
Imbolc, 10–11
Imposter syndrome, 100
alleviating the effects of,
100–101
Incantation, 264, 267
Indifference, healing, 182–183
Injustices, protecting those
faced with, 184–185
Intentions, 267
setting clear, powerful,
21, 39
Intolerance, healing lingering,
186–187
Isolation, healing feelings of,
198–199

J

Jars, 27
Jasmine, in getting better
sleep, 72
Jasper, 32
in alignment of mind and
body, 130, 132
in assuaging anger, 83, 84
in being accepted for
authentic identities,
163, 164
in healing apathy, 238
in healing broken heart,
89, 90

in healing feelings of
isolation, 198, 199
in healing negative
responses, 123
prior to lovemaking, 68
in restoring trees, 242
in revealing authentic self,
56, 57
in shining protective
energy into home, 215
in struggling with mental
health, 159
Jealousy, 78
release from petty, 108–109
Jojoba oil
in boosting your healing
strength, 96–97
in creating cohesion
between groups and
community, 200
Journaling, 9
in disconnecting with
universe, 116
Joy
bringing into home,
221–222
in celebratory living, 16

K

Kitchen witch, 19
Knowing thyself, 8
Knowledge, commitment
to, 15

L

Lammas, 10–11
Last quarter moon, 15
Lavender (Lavandula
angustifolia), 29, 34
in aiding conception, 60
in being accepted for
authentic identities, 163
in creation of home
sanctuary, 227
in enhancing receptivity to
psychic messages, 117
in foot soak in summoning
forgiveness, 133
in fostering patience, 106,
107
in getting better sleep, 72
in getting past being stuck
in the past, 169, 170
in healing home of
unwelcoming vibes, 207
in healing self-doubt,
190, 191

Lavender (cont.)
in improving
concentration, 102
in making healing poppets,
147
in recovering from
addiction, 167, 168
in reducing stress, 87
in release from jealousy,
108, 109
Lavender oil
in cleansing air, 248
in creation of home
sanctuary, 227, 228
in healing home of
unwelcoming vibes, 207
in healing intolerance, 186
in healing negative
responses, 123
in healing weakness in
psychic abilities, 119–120
in renewing heart to
possibility of, 111
in renewing spirit from
negative energies, 139
in soothing spirit, 219
Learning, commitment to, 15
Lemon juice
in healing common cold,
70
in healing impurities in
drinking water, 246, 247
in healing negative
energies, 211–212
Lemon oil
in beating fatigue, 52
in getting energy boost, 52
Leo, 13
Lethargic effects, combating
and healing, 158–159
Libra, 13
Life's moments, magickal
value in celebrating, 16
Light, healing for Earth,
261–262
Litha, 10–11
"Lone wolf" attitudes, healing,
188–189
Longevity, healing body of
energy that dampens,
156–157
Love
healing power of
intentional, 78
renewing heart to
possibility of, 111–112
Loved ones, easing anxieties
of your, 153
Lovemaking, 68–69

M

Mabon, 10–11
Macrocosm, 17
Magick
defined, 7
individual versus
sympathy, 24
Magickal workings, goal of,
206
Meditation, 9, 20–21, 40
Memory, improving your,
92–93
Mental health, 16
struggles with, 159–160
Microcosm, 17
Mind
alignment with body,
130–132
drawing calming vibes to
the anxious, 81–82
healing your, 78–109
Mint (Mentha), 29
in building a witch's ladder,
230
in creating happy and
optimistic energy,
94, 95
in designating natural
wonders as national
parks, 250, 251
emanating into cooking,
232
in healing impurities in
drinking water, 246
in healing low energy, 178
in healing righteousness,
141
Moon cycle, casting off
disappointments,
192–193
Moons, 14–15
phases of, 37
relationship with, 17
Moon water elixir, creating
healing, 66–67, 139
Moore, Thomas, 235
Mortar and pestle, 34, 267
Myers-Briggs test, 9, 268

N

Names, writing in book of
love, 171–172
Natural cycles, alignment
with, 113–114
Natural wonders, designating
as national parks and
wildlife preserves,
250–251

Nature, connection to, 9–12
Negative, toxic patterns,
healing from, 98–99
Negative energy
being proactive about, 218
creation of black salt in
healing, 223–224
pentagram in dispersing,
150
renewing spirit from,
139–140
stovetop boil in purifying
home's air, 211–212
New moon, 14
length of, 213–214
in recovering from
addiction, 168
Nutmeg (Myristica fragrans),
30
in healing discord, 176
in reducing stress, 87
Nutrition, maintaining better,
54–55

O

Oceans, healing of, 254–255
Orange oil
for body positivity, 76
in celebrating
achievements, 194
in charging your crystals,
47
in creating happy and
optimistic energy, 94
in creating witchy bell
charm, 209
in healing home of clutter,
213
in healing "lone wolf"
attitudes, 188
in healing self-doubt, 165
in improving
concentration, 102
in lifting depression, 85
in reducing stress, 87
in struggling with mental
health, 159
in summoning confidence
and courage, 137
Orange slices, in bringing joy
into home, 221–222
Oregano (Origanum vulgare),
28
in alleviating effects of
imposter syndrome, 100
in assuaging anger, 83, 84
in cleansing air, 248
in harnessing healing
power of, 225, 226

in releasing unrealistic
expectations, 104, 105
Ostara, 10–11

P

Pain, drawing energy of, from
the body, 58–59
Parsley (*Petroselinum crispum*), 29
in cleansing energy
blockages, 236
in clearing body of energy
that dampens longevity,
156, 157
in creating sigils, 174
in drawing pain from body,
58, 59
in giving magickal
protection to spirit, 121
in healing from grief, 154
in healing regions affected
by food security, 244
in preventing illness, 50
Past, getting stuck in the,
169–170
Pentagram, 268
creating in healing
indifference, 183
in dispersing negative
energies, 150
drawing in fostering
patience, 107
in healing oceans, 254–255
healing power of garden
plants in creating,
225–226
in shining protective
energy into home, 215
Pepper, in creation of black
salt, 223
Peppercorn, in healing from
negative, toxic patterns,
98–99
Peppermint oil, 34
in beating fatigue, 52
in drawing strength to
work, 217
in getting energy boost, 52
in healing common cold,
70
in healing Earth from
floods, 256
in healing home of clutter,
213
in improving
concentration, 102
in recovering from
addiction, 167
in relieving tension
headaches, 62

Pessimism, releasing, 233–234
Pisces, 13
Planet, healing the, 235–265
Playing cards, in building a
witch's ladder, 230
Poppets, 268
power of, in sending
healing vibes to friends
and family, 147–148
Potions, 23, 268
Power, stepping into your, 24
Praxis, 15, 268
smoke divination, 123–124
Psychic abilities, healing
weakness in your,
119–120
Psychic message, enhancing
spirit's receptivity to,
117–118
Pumpkin, carving healing
symbols into, 261–262

Q

Quartz. *See* Clear quartz;
Rose quartz; Smoky
quartz

R

Righteousness, embracing
healing, 141–142
Ritual knife, 27
Rituals, 23, 45, 46, 268
Rosemary oil
in beating fatigue, 52
for body positivity, 76
in getting energy boost, 52
in healing common cold,
70
Rosemary (*Rosmarinus officinalis*), 26, 29
in aiding conception, 60
in boosting your healing
strength, 96–97
in bringing joy into home,
221, 222
in building a witch's ladder,
229, 231
in cleansing air, 248
in cleansing energy
blockages, 236
in creation of home
sanctuary, 227
in enhancing receptivity to
psychic messages, 117
in fostering patience, 106,
107
in harnessing healing
power of, 225, 226

in healing ego weaknesses,
180, 181
in healing energy
interference, 196
in healing low energy, 178
in healing negative
energies, 211
in healing oceans, 254
in healing self-doubt,
190, 191
in helping committed
relationships through
rough patches, 151, 152
in infusing energy of love
and healing, 171, 172
in preventing illness, 50
prior to lovemaking, 68
Rose quartz, 32
for body positivity, 76
in building a witch's ladder,
230
in celebrating
achievements, 194
in creation of home
sanctuary, 227, 228
emanating into cooking,
232
in healing broken heart,
89, 91
in healing energy
interference, 196
in healing feelings of
isolation, 198
in lifting depression, 85, 86
in making healing poppets,
147, 148
prior to lovemaking, 68
in renewing spirit from
negative energies, 139
in struggling with mental
health, 159

S

Sabbats, 9–11
Sachets, 268
in giving magickal
protection to your
spirit, 121–122
in helping recovery from
surgery, 149–150
in preventing illness, 51
Sage (*Salvia officinalis*), 29
in aiding conception, 60
in cleansing air, 248
in drawing calming vibes
to the anxious mind, 81
in enhancing receptivity to
psychic messages, 117
in getting better sleep, 72

Sage (cont.)
  in giving magickal
    protection to spirit, 121
  in harnessing healing
    power of, 225, 226
  in healing impurities in
    drinking water, 246
  in healing negative
    energies, 211
  in making healing poppets,
    147
  in protecting against
    injustices, 184
  in summoning confidence
    and courage, 137
Sagittarius, 13
Salt, 26
Salubrious, intentional living,
  15–16
Samhain, 9, 10–11
Sanctuary, creation of, in
  home, 227–228
Scorpio, 13
Seashells, in building a witch's
  ladder, 230
Self, connection to, 8–9
Self-doubt, healing, 165–166,
  190–191
Self-growth, 15
Sigils, 268
  creating, 174–175
Sleep, better, 72–73
Smoke
  in cleaning air, 248–249
  healing negative responses
    and, 123–125
Smoky quartz, 32
  in aiding conception, 60
  in foot soak in summoning
    forgiveness, 133
  in getting better sleep, 72
  in healing common cold,
    70, 71
  in healing Earth from
    wildfire, 257, 258
  in healing from grief, 154
  in healing from guilt, 128
  in healing "lone wolf"
    attitudes, 188
  in lifting depression, 85
  in preventing illness, 50
  in reducing stress, 87, 88
Social media, advent of, 20
Sodalite, 32
  in alignment of mind and
    body, 130, 131
  in being accepted for
    authentic identities,
    163, 164

in healing broken heart,
  89, 90
in healing discord, 176
in healing from guilt, 128
in healing righteousness,
  141
in healing weakness in
  psychic abilities, 119, 120
in making healing poppets,
  147, 148
in repairing friendships, 161
in shining protective
  energy into home,
  215, 216
Solitary witches, 19–20
Spellcraft, methods used in,
  35–36
Spells, 45, 46
  aligning timing of, 37
  aligning with cosmic
    energy, 12
  casting, 23, 268
Spellwork cleanup, 42
Spices, 29–30
Spirit
  healing of your, 110–142
  magickal protection to
    your, 121–122
  soothing your, 219–220
Spiritual rut, healing from,
  126–127
Star anise
  in bringing joy into home,
    221, 222
  in easing anxieties of loved
    ones, 153
Stars, relationship with, 17
Stress ball, in reducing stress,
  87–88
Sun, 12
Sweet orange oil, 33
  in repairing friendships, 161
Symbols for the elements, 36
Sympathy magick, 146, 268

T

Tarot cards, in building a
  witch's ladder, 230
Taurus, 13
Tea tree oil, 34
  in being proactive about
    negative energy, 218
  in boosting your healing
    strength, 96
  in healing discord, 176
  in healing intolerance, 186
  in making healing poppets,
    147

in overcoming lingering
  illness, 64
Tension headaches, relieving,
  62–63
Third eye, 118, 131, 268
Thyme (Thymus vulgaris), 29
  in alleviating effects of
    imposter syndrome, 100
  in being accepted for
    authentic identities, 163
  in boosting your healing
    strength, 96
  in charging your crystals,
    47
  in cleansing energy
    blockages, 236
  in drawing strength to
    work, 217
  in enhancing receptivity to
    psychic messages, 117
  in fostering patience, 106,
    107
  in harnessing healing
    power of, 225
  in healing righteousness,
    141
  in healing self-doubt,
    190, 191
  in recovering from
    addiction, 167, 168
  in sachet in recovering
    from surgery, 149
  in summoning confidence
    and courage, 137, 138
Tools, 34–35
Tourmaline, 32
  in assuaging anger, 83, 84
  in being proactive about
    negative energy, 218
  in celebrating
    achievements, 194
  in drawing pain from body,
    58, 59
  in healing from grief, 154
  in healing home of clutter,
    213
  in overcoming lingering
    illness, 64
  in preventing illness, 50
  in protecting against
    injustices, 184
  in sachet in recovering
    from surgery, 149
  in summoning confidence
    and courage, 137
Transformation, 15
Trees, restoring and
  bolstering health of
  worldwide, 242–243

THE HEALING POWER OF WITCHCRAFT

Triple Goddess, 74
Turmeric (*Curcuma longa*), 30
   in healing Earth from
      floods, 256
   in healing from negative,
      toxic patterns, 98–99
   in healing indifference, 182
   in revealing authentic self,
      56, 57

U

Universe
   disconnecting with, 115–116
   governing of, 7
   parts to, 9
   in witchcraft, 7

V

Vanilla oil in getting better
   sleep, 72
Vibes
   emanating healing, into
      cooking, 232
   healing home of
      unwelcoming, 207–208
Virgo, 13

W

Waning crescent, 15
   in healing broken heart, 91
Waning gibbous, 15
Water, 22, 36
   healing impurities in
      drinking, 246–247
Waxing crescent, 14
Waxing gibbous, 14
Waxing moon, in healing
   broken heart, 90
Wheel of the Year, 9, 268
White candles, 26
Widdershins, 99, 268
Wildfire, healing Earth from,
   257–258
Wildlife preserves,
   designating national
   wonders as, 250–251
Witchcraft
   creatrix, 250, 267
   defined, 7
   empathetic, sympathetic
      nature of, 205
   essential tools of, 26–27
   guiding principles of, 8–17
   healing power of, 7
   path to, 17–18

Witches
   building ladder, 229–231
   calling to action, 145
   color of door, 207–208
   goals of, 15
   home of, 206
   innate ability to perform
      healing magick, 5
   reverence and connection
      to nature, 235
   selecting your mode, 23
   solitary, 19–20
   spirit of, 110
   states of mind, 20–21
   types of, 18–19
   understanding own
      intuition and intents, 5
   in witchcraft, 7
Witches' New Year, 9
Work, drawing strength and
   concentration to, 217
World, healing your, 204–265
Wortcunning/cunning, 70,
   268

Y

Ylang-ylang oil, 34
   in celebrating
      achievements, 194
   in connecting group with
      healing prayers, 202
   in designating natural
      wonders as national
      parks, 250
   in getting better sleep, 72
   in helping committed
      relationships through
      rough patches, 151
   in improving
      concentration, 102
   in lifting depression, 85
   prior to lovemaking, 68
   in reducing stress, 87
Yoga, 9
Yule, 10–11

Z

Zodiac chart, 12

ACKNOWLEDGMENTS

I will be forever grateful for the energies that aligned to make this book a reality, and those energies are embodied in my support system. Manifestation work is a group effort, and I am fortunate enough to be surrounded by the best.

To my husband, Mike, you sweeten the victories, soften the disappointments, steady the wheel, and love endlessly. Thank you for healing me each and every day. You are my original magick moment.

To my children, Grayson and Jack, may you know a healed world. May you always lift others up and always know you can come home to ground. May you light the way but hold space for the dark. May you grow strong and be a force for good. Mama loves you.

To my parents, it is because of your foundation, your love, your abundance, and the beautiful life you two have built together that I am here, unafraid to claim my life path as a witch. I can't think of a better parenting goal than creating an environment for my own children that will allow them to live their truest, most authentic, happiest self; you have achieved that tenfold. Thank you, God bless you, and I love you.

To Kathy, Michelle, and Mike, I am so grateful for our madness. Thank you for being in my beautiful people clubhouse.

To my friends, especially the Madmoms, KNC, Knotties, Grampa Dave, Natalie, Skelly, Laura, and even Spike. Your love, laughter, and support have made for a lifetime of invaluable adventures, lessons, and memories. Oh yeah, all right, take it easy, baby, make it last all night.

To my witchy support system, especially Louisa, Briony, and Josie. You witches make my heart sing with real magick.

And for the entire Witch With Me community, you inspire me endlessly.

To my team at Penguin Random House, you are simply the best. Meg Ilasco, Debbie Reyhan, and especially Susan Randol. Thank you for guiding this "green" witch through the process and pushing this book to where it needed to be in order to help heal the world.

To Gran E, Nanny, Poppop, Aunt Helen, and Holmie. I feel you with me always. I hope I make you proud.

ABOUT THE AUTHOR

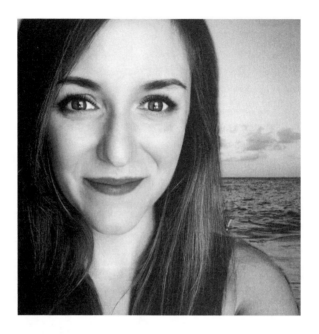

MEG ROSENBRIAR is a practicing hedgewitch with a focus on healing energy work, herbalism, tarot, yoga, numerology, and embracing an intentional, witchy lifestyle. She has been a student of spirituality her whole life with a degree in Religious Studies from Merrimack College and a Master of Arts from Yale University School of Divinity. She is the cofounder of Witch With Me, a community platform by witches for witches dedicated to discovering, honoring, preserving, and sharing authentic witchcraft. Meg resides with her husband and two sons on the Connecticut shoreline.

Hi there,

We hope you enjoyed reading *The Healing Power of Witchcraft*. If you have any questions or concerns about your book, please contact **customerservice@penguinrandomhouse.com** so we can take care of them. We're here and happy to help.

Also, please consider writing a review on your favorite retailer's website to let others know what you thought of the book and to help them with their buying decision.

Sincerely,
Zeitgeist Publishing